# *The Blessing of Sarah*

## MOROLAYO ANNE OWOPUTI

authorHOUSE®

AuthorHouse™ UK Ltd.
500 Avebury Boulevard
Central Milton Keynes, Mk9 2BE
www.authorhouse.co.uk
Phone: 08001974150

To share your testimonies with the Author or for ministration, call
+234 902 020 2100, morolayo2020@gmail.com
twitter handle: @mowoputi

First published by AuthorHouse 2009

ISBN: 978-1-5176-8105-0

This book is printed on acid-free paper.

Printed in the United Kingdom

All scriptures of the Bible quoted in this book are from KJV and NKJV

And I will bless her, and give you a son from her!
Yea I will bless her, and she shall become a mother of nations;
kings of people shall be from her

- Genesis 17:16p

Daughter, you are blessed! Go and conceive in this light

**Bishop David Oyedepo,**
*President, Living Faith Ministries, Otta, Nigeria.*

It's a powerful, powerful, powerful book!

**Rev. Sam Adeyemi,**
*Senior Pastor, Daystar Christian Centre, Lagos, Nigeria.*

I know this is of God! It's a reversal of what the enemy is putting on women.

**Bryan Pullinger**
*President, Brian Pullinger Networking for Revival, UK*

I love this book! It offers real hope and faith for those desiring to have a baby.

**Linda Knox**
*Host, Reaching out through Compassionate Caring (ROTCC), USA.*

In the beginning, "And the Lord God *formed* man"
*- Genesis 2:7*

And the Lord God said "I have *formed* you"
*- Isaiah 44:21b*

More so "I *formed* you from the *Womb* "
*- Isaiah 44:2a, 24a and 49:5a*

In fact, "Before I *formed* you in the *Womb* I knew you"
*- Jeremiah 1:5*

**This book is therefore dedicated to all women**

Whose babies will be *formed* in their *Wombs*, notwithstanding.

# CONTENTS

# Author's Inspiration

This book was inspired by a series of recurring event I have witnessed over the years. Early on in my life I realized that I always felt moved with compassion toward people who are suffering. I always wished I had a supernatural power to help them come out of their agonizing predicaments and sufferings. As I grew older and attended church services, I heard many preachers teach about a God in heaven who is our creator and who has astonishing power to accomplish wondrous things in the lives of humans. I heard many testimonies to this power!

I then set out to search out the truth of these teachings myself. So I began studying my Bible judiciously, as though I would be required to write a professional examination on it, because I was eager to verify the "facts" presented in these numerous sermons about this God's power. In the course of this intensive study of my Bible, I made a remarkable discovery: The facts were real and not a fairy tale.

As I followed the teachings in the Word and learnt how to pray for those people towards whom my heart was compassionate—to see therein the interplay of human drama and divine involvement—I saw this God's power working in and changing them for the better and turning their lives around. Above all, I saw this same God's power working tremendously in my own life and affairs and always moving me ahead of my peers to an uncommon *next level.* So it was that a university friend of mine who witnessed the undeniable proofs of working of God's power in my life once asked me, "Are you the only one who is serving God? Why is it that you are always and consistently getting results?"

Indeed, this consistent experience of what God's power can accomplish in human life led me to intensify my prayers that He might showcase more of this power over the affairs of men. I realized that most of my prayers were directed towards potential mothers (and especially expectant mothers), and both then and now my heart never ceases to be moved by them. The most interesting thing about this is that, as I pray and believe God for known loved ones waiting on God for the fruit of the womb, before I know it, He shows me in dreams that they shall soon conceive, and shortly after I see them become pregnant and bear their babies. For instance, there was a time He showed me in a vision sequentially, two of my aunts who had been waiting for almost half a decade to bear a child being heavily pregnant. On seeing this, I knew God was at work. Few months later, one of them visited the house and as she was about discussing with my mum, I quickly related the event to her and in awe, she said, " .....exactly what I came to tell mum" that she was few months pregnant. Not too long again, I was able to see my second aunt and narrated the event to her seeing her pregnant. She then responded with a hug and said "I am actually pregnant" after waiting these years.

These experience and many more have given me the courage to turn aside like Moses, who changed his position out of curiosity to understand why the bush was burning yet not consumed. There must be a message in the recurring event of seeing expectant mothers bear after being blessed to see it in a dream even before they conceived. It was a real eye-opener to discover, after I had moved out of the environment where I frequently saw expectant loved ones that the dreams about some of them getting pregnant still persisted! I still have these dreams and not long after receive the wonderful news that another woman was either pregnant or had just dedicated her baby. Having witnessed this repeatedly, I can attest that these dreams are not mere ordinary occurrences happening by chance.

Then I asked the custodian of this power—God—what He was up to in allowing me to see these events in a dream before any eye sees the physical babies. While still waiting for an answer, my prayer life focused on seeing God's game plan for such a time as this for expectant mothers. Then not too long after, I heard in my spirit: "The Blessing of Sarah" *What! This is strange!* I know "the blessing of Abraham" *but not... of Sarah.*

All these questions were swirling about in my mind when He opened up my understanding and explained this mystery. Yet I was overwhelmed by this exposition. So in order to help me comprehend the intended message better, in laymen's language, He showed me repeatedly in my dreams a vision of Dr. David Oyedepo beckoning me to come. Whenever I woke up from one of these dreams, I asked Him: "Why this vision of Dr. David Oyedepo at this time? What about him, Lord?"

Then I heard the response: "Hook up with him online." Therefore, for the first time, I went online to watch the services of the Winners Chapel in Otta, Nigeria, including archive services, and that was it!

My head and heart were opened to the mystery of what He was explaining to me all this time about the blessing of Sarah. I was shown this mystery in graphic images as I watched some members come bearing their babies in their arms to testify how they had waited for a baby—some for a decade or longer. I was astounded by these "live" testimonies from no fewer than 20 women sharing their exceptional testimonies of how God's power had brought the blessing of a baby out of barrenness.

My faith abounded as I was presented with testimony after testimony of God's power over barrenness. At this juncture, knowing that this was not a figment of my imagination, I determined to present this mystery in a book. That is how *The Blessing of Sarah*, which you are reading now, came to be.

Finally, let me say that I consider it a rare privilege to be given this assignment, because, on the basis of human standards and natural experience alone, I am not qualified to handle this task, but by His Spirit working in me, and by the inspiration of the Almighty, I have not only understood the lessons He revealed to me but done justice to it adequately. Therefore, without exception, this book is a must–read for all expecting couples, potential couples, and all young ladies out there who expect one day to be married and bear kids. It is a packed resource also for pregnant women, craving to experience *full time* gestation period without miscarriage; and anticipate to have a normal childbirth. In short, there is a blessing in it for all categories of women that desire to bear children in their lifetime and without trouble too. Even if you do not have an earthly mother, please do not despair; rather look at Sarah your mother as she is presented in this book.

# CHAPTER ONE

### The Famous Blessings of Abraham and the "Unknown" Blessing of Sarah

*And I will bless her, and give you a son from her! Yea, I will bless her, and she shall*

*become a mother of nations; kings of people shall be from her*

*- Genesis 17:16p*

| |
|---|
| *Promises, however, are God's intentions for the future of man* |

Down to this very day the story of Abraham is very famous throughout the world. Even pagan cultures have once heard about this affluent patriarch whose status and wealth are beyond dispute. It was obvious even to the spiritually-blind eyes in his own days that Abraham was an embodiment of blessing. Abraham is a figurative expression of wealth and prosperity. Students of the Bible know that he is the father of blessings and nations to this very day. God blessed this man and made his name great so that even today we believe so much how

1

Abraham's blessing are ours, and how this blessing makes us blessed in the morning and in the evening. The story of Abraham's blessing began in Genesis 12 when God instructed him to move to a new land and promised to bless him there. And God certainly did bless him, as recorded in Genesis 13:2, and Abraham became very rich in livestock and in silver and gold.

Abraham was incredibly wealthy. For instance, about 318 servants were born and reared in Abraham's house (Genesis 14:14), which means that he was also taking care of the parents of those servants who were living in his house. Abraham was so rich that he despaired collecting even a strand of other people's thread to add to his own belongings so as to prevent any human being's claim that he had made Abraham rich. In short, Abraham was greatly blessed. And so we were taught from childhood, even before many of us came to know Christ as Lord and Savior, that Abraham's blessing are ours and that we are the sons and daughters of Father Abraham. We sing it in the children's church, and confess it in the adult church. We pray it, we mutter it, and our pastors teach us so much about it because they want us to be blessed and experience that same blessing. So we see that Abraham's blessing extend to our own day. I believe in the blessing of Abraham and the fact that we are his seed and that he is the father of all blessing.

Despite the fact that Abraham was blessed and never lacked a thing he wanted, still he was not satisfied. God gave him all the physical and material blessing he desired and even intangible blessing of promises, yet Abraham was not fulfilled, for there was one thing that God had not given to him. So one day Abraham summoned the courage (because Abraham feared God) to ask God for an additional blessing. In Genesis 15:2, he asked "What will You give me?"

What an ironic statement? Despite all he had been given, in both tangible and intangible substance, Abraham asked God, "What will you give me?" He proceeded to ask God for a child. This implies that Abraham needed an additional blessing in order to crown his blessing and bring it to fullness. I like Abraham's request of God because he was giving God a strong reason why he could not simply be satisfied with all of his other blessings because he had not received the crowning blessing—a child. God was delighted with this question because He had been waiting for Abraham to ask it so that He could gradually unfold to him the mystery of the blessing of Sarah. So God's response to Abraham was that his children would be innumerable as the stars in heaven, and therefore Abraham believed God such that it was registered for him in the book of records as a righteous act according to Genesis 15:2-6. When Abraham looked up, what he saw were you and I that would come to earth someday; therefore it was recounted for him as an act of faith because he believed.

God took it even further by telling Abraham how He would make provision for the land that his descendants would inherit and occupy, and Abraham believed all that God spoke to him about on this great day. Promises, however, are God's intentions for the future of man, and whenever they are not forthcoming, we humans have a tendency to easily forget about the intangible substance of promises and settle for the tangible alternatives. The Bible does not tell us how old Abraham was when God spoke these words to him. Let us assume he was in his 70s or early 80s, and that after waiting several decades for God's promises of children, Abraham began to consider the visions through which this promise was given to him as a mere illusion, nothing more than wishful dreams that arose from nothing more than his own human desires. As a result, he began to exercise fear as God's introductory speech to him on this matter was a cautioning "Fear not, Abram: I am thy shield and thy exceeding great reward" according to Genesis 15:1(KJV). God could see in Abram a fear of the unknown which culminates from the fact that he was fast approaching the centenarian class (100 years old) still without a child.

This same thing happens to many of us even today in various areas of our lives. God has given us promises in words, in dreams, in visions by night and day, has spoken to us through His servants and prophets. Perhaps He has even used repetitive and sequential events to communicate to us that His promises are *yes and Amen,* to convince us that He cannot go back on His word nor change as He will bring His promises to pass in our lives according to His plan for our lives. Yet, despite all that assurance, we seem unsatisfied with invisible promises without visible results. So before long, we begin to downplay these promises as though they were never made to us and begin to pursue alternatives out of fear.

Abraham the father of faith sought an alternative and so made a mistake at first by sleeping with a handmaid at the request of Sarah. He did so without hesitation. He did not even try to convince Sarah of the fact that God had already promised him that they would have children and thus she should not encourage him to commit this sin of unbelief against God, who made the

4

promise and called him righteous for believing it. Instead, Abraham went in and lay with the woman and she became pregnant. This was proof that the infertility problem lay not with Abraham but with Sarah even though God already planned to bless Abraham through Sarah and not Hagar.

God was not pleased with Abraham because of this act. Heaven was silent on Abraham for thirteen years. Abraham was eighty six years old when Ishmael was born going by Gen 16:16; and he was ninety-nine years when again God appeared to him according to Genesis 17:1 telling him to walk before Him and be blameless. In saying this, we can infer that God no longer saw Abraham as blameless as he used to be and was now reminding him to be blameless before Him. God reminded Abraham that His promises of multiplying Abraham's descendants exceedingly was still potent and had not changed despite the fact that Abraham seemed to have brushed it aside.

Abraham admitted his wrongdoing and fearing that he had compromised his faith by no longer waiting on the promise but instead seeking alternatives, immediately fell on his face. This happens often when we are walking with God but decide that His timing is off or at best too slow.

*Delayed blessing can make us to act on our own will or ways*

Delayed blessing can make us to act on our own will or ways. Because His timing is entirely different from our own timing we become impatient having to wait for so long and so seek alternatives to escape living in uncertainty. We see that in spite of this mistake God yet extended His love to Abraham. He renewed and reinforced His promises to him—this time by explaining to him in clearer terms how He would bless Abraham and Sarah with children.

At this point, let's pause and think a little about this last statement. You will quite agree with me that the understanding of a matter could aid in waiting and continuing to work towards achieving a desired result. It can be very frustrating when God tells us, repeatedly and consistently, that He will do something for us without telling us *how* He will do it. Oftentimes, we become weary in waiting. Many times, even though God gives us a word of assurance with a date without mentioning the year that He will bring His pronounced promises to pass, we begin to look for logical alternatives when everything around is not confirming the possibility of its happening. This is because we are kept in the dark and cannot catch a glimpse of how it could happen—and may even begin to doubt that such an impossibility could occur at all in this day and age. We must learn to ask God guiding questions to travel through whenever we do not understand how we will be able to exercise patience till God's promises become a reality in our lives. Then we will eventually be able to testify that He is Lord over the very matters that once troubled us.

Think of this example. If you tell a 40-year-old man who stands four feet tall that he will become six feet tall by month end without informing him as to how you intend to accomplish this seemingly impossible task (i.e., adding two feet to his height), what is he likely to do? The rational man will try to make logical sense of the matter using his fundamental knowledge of human biology to analyze how this could be possible. A man who understands the medical implications of what you are telling him will not admit its possibility unless you explain to him carefully—after the fashion of his biology teacher—how adding two feet to his height is possible. If you do not do this, the man will dismiss such promises and instead seek possible alternatives, if there are any. Understanding is vital. It is key to our walk with God. We must understand His ways as well as His acts. He wants to show us things and assists us understand better so we can get the best and not settle for less.

The way God walks with man is based on man's understanding of His ways through the day–to–day dealings between God and man. Let's say God tells you He will give you bread tomorrow. According to *His* timing the bread will arrive on your doorstep by 8 p.m. If He does not disclose the timing to you, you will probably go and buy bread by 6 p.m. or 7 p.m. when you do not see the bread He promised; thinking that perhaps you misunderstood Him or that He had changed His mind. But if He had told you the exact time–8 p.m.–you would wait, no matter how hungry you were, knowing well that His own bread would more than compensate for all your long hours of waiting for His bread to arrive.

God knows from the thoughts of our hearts whether we will eventually go and buy the bread before 8 p.m. The man who buys the bread at 7 p.m. (because he does not receive the bread when he wanted it) would have thought about it before then. He would have thought, *if the bread doesn't get here by suppertime, I'm going to just go buy a loaf.*

Once we fail the test, God will set another one for us because He is interested in our growth while walking with Him so that we might mature to the fullness of the stature He desires for us. Abraham could not wait, despite his numerous encounters with God and the fact that he was even a man who spoke with God and was a friend of God. He was not immune to this syndrome common to all men of seeking alternatives to God's promises. Abraham was not exempt from this doubt because God had not finished unfolding to him how He intended to bring His promise of giving them children to pass. Abraham could not pass the test until God fully explained to him how He would do it. God wants to give each of us the level of understanding that will not only give us immunity against seeking alternatives during our time of waiting but that will show us how our long-expected miracles will reach our hand.

# Scriptural Notes

- Genesis 12: 1-3

- Genesis 13:2

- Genesis 14: 14

- Genesis 15: 1

- Genesis 15:2-6

- Genesis 16: 16

- Genesis 17: 1

# CHAPTER TWO

*The Blessing of Sarah*

*And I will bless her, and give you a son from her! Yea, I will bless her, and she shall become a mother of nations; kings of people shall be from her*

*- Genesis 17:16p*

> *It is the blessing that enables you to conceive and bear a child, no matter what the medical verdict is*

We have seen how Abraham, the father of faith, settled for an alternative that he could touch and see that yielded immediate result without requiring him to wait any longer. Abraham and Sarah looked for a way to solve the problem based on their own understanding. This was not pleasing to God. God did not forsake Him, however, but rather came to help Abraham understand His ways regarding this matter. This is the very theme of this book: God wants to show many people in our day how He intends to bring to pass the child-bearing promises He made to each one. He has told you in His Word that you shall be fruitful and countless times he has reiterated it to you through every communication medium available to get it across to you. Perhaps some friends and loved ones at times have told you they could see you pregnant and having your baby's dedication. Pastors and prophets presiding over you might also have given you a word of assurance on countless occasions and shared how God has assured them that you will conceive and bear a baby. Yet nothing is happening ... and you are beginning to doubt the authenticity of their calling.

Perhaps you have also fasted and prayed and given sacrifices and even made some gigantic vows to God just to move Him to action, yet you do not conceive. Abram had the same experience. He had heard God tell him several times that he would be a father of many nations and had seen God show him how numerous his seed (descendants) would be–like the stars of heaven. God had even showed him the land his seed would inherit and occupy and given him assurance by cutting a covenant with him that he would become a father of many nations and that kings would arise from his line, but Abram was yet to see the fulfillment of any of these promises and assurances. He had waited for decades and there was no sign of the blessing.

So Abram sought an alternative, and God had to remind him to walk before him blameless so as to see the glory that God had promised him. God also changed Abram's name to Abraham to reflect his new status as a father of nations and reassured him in Genesis17:6 "I will make you *exceedingly fruitful*; and I will make nations of you, and kings shall come from you."

But so as not to keep Abraham in perpetual darkness about the delayed fulfillment of the promise, God gave Abraham a clue. He told him in Genesis 17:16 that the way He would make Abraham the father of nations was through the blessing of Sarah. In effect He says, "I will bless Sarah and also give you a son by her which will make you become exceedingly fruitful like I have told you earlier. Yea, I will bless her, and she shall be a mother of nations that will cause you to become a father of nations and kings of people shall come from her, which is the promise I have already given to you."

In a nutshell, God was explaining to Abraham that it would come to pass through His blessing upon Sarah—the human with a womb—that would make Abraham—the human without the womb—exceedingly fruitful and a father of nations and kings. So we see that it was blessing of Sarah that made Abraham become a father of nations and of kings, whereas it was the blessing of Abraham that made Abraham exceedingly prosperous. When God created all living creatures that move on the earth according to Genesis 1:1-22, He did not leave them without the blessing. Despite the fact that God looked at all of these creatures He had made and saw that they were good, He never just left them to mere goodness without the blessing that would enable them to fulfill the purpose for which there were created. Thus in Genesis 1:22, God blessed them, implying that they should be exceedingly fruitful and multiply and fill the earth.

God blessed all living creatures with reproduction, which in this context, is the impartation to reproduce its kind. God pronounced the same blessing upon the human beings He created in His very own image to enable them to become fruitful.

God blessed them with the blessing of reproduction according to His plan for creating them. That is why to this very day it is exceedingly rare to find an animal that is barren or impotent: in fact it is practically impossible because the blessing is working on them. So ask, "Why then is barrenness present in human beings?"

As you read on, you will discover how barrenness crept into the human race and woman—the human with the womb—for in the beginning it was not so.

### Your case is certainly not as bad as Sarah's

Perhaps many cases of human barrenness stem from the fact that we are yet to engage the blessing of Sarah in the same way that we consciously engage the blessing of Abraham vis-a-vis our finances. The blessing of Sarah is incomprehensible to physicians, and it suspends all biological mechanisms that would prevent a woman from conceiving and bearing a child. Sarah's barrenness is the longest case of barrenness recorded in history. *So take heart!* Sarah had even passed menopause. She was 90 years old! No woman on earth has broken Sarah's world record of waiting for the promise of child. Your case is certainly not as bad as Sarah's. Thus you shall soon conceive because no one will have to wait for that long again for the fulfillment of the promise. As you digest the unraveled secrets in this book, in faith I can assure you by the anointing of the Holy One that you will conceive and bring forth sons and daughters by the Spirit of the Lord.

*So what is this "blessing of Sarah" all about?* Why have we heard only about the blessing of Abraham and not about the blessing of

Sarah? The story all began in Genesis, the book of beginnings. In Genesis 11:30, the Bible tells us that Sarai, Abram's wife, was barren because she had no child. Meanwhile, Sarai's husband, Abram is a friend of God and God is interested in him; and all that pertains to him including Sarai; though she was yet to be grafted into His covenant to him. God disclosed His plans to Abram, who enjoyed obeying God and seeing His plans fulfilled. In Abram's walk with God, he understood how God had been leading him to obtain his possessions and dealing with him in making him prosperous. Abram believed and knew that the blessing that God pronounced upon him in Genesis 12:2-3 were real and were working for him because he could see himself moving from one level of advancement to another. He knew he had been imparted to become exalted, and his humanity empowered to magnetise wealth, riches, and favors to him. What's more, Abram could see how God was always fighting for him plaguing all who sought to tamper with his belongings, including Sarai. Abram was so conscious about the working of the blessing upon his life that he rejected king's offer to make him richer because he understood that God's blessing on him would give him a hundredfold what any man was able to give him. So Abram did not add other people's belongings to his own, so that it would be glaringly evident that the blessings of God alone had made Abram rich and nothing more.

Abram could not, however, act in the same manner when it came to the issue of his having a child. When Sarai told him to go into her maid Hagar, Abram did not hesitate, nor did he decline lest people say it was his servants who had given him an heir and that the child born to him by servants would be the inheritor of all the possessions God had given him. Abram never said any of these things; he just heeded the voice of Sarai straight away and went in unto Hagar.

Some Bible scholars have suggested that Abram heeded Sarai's request without questioning to get relief from her nagging. But if that were the case, I believe the Bible would have recorded that Sarah was nagging Abram or making their home-life unbearable because she wanted a child. Just as the Bible records Hannah's complaint and vehement cries to her husband (1 Samuel 1:8) and Rachel's lament "give me children or else I die" (Genesis 30: 1), so we would have learned of Sarai's anguish and nagging if it had been so. Moreover, as it was recorded of how that Sarai dealt harshly with her maid Hagar until she fled from her presence (Genesis 16:6); it would have been written too if she had dealt with Abram in like manner. Sarai likewise seemed to be a woman of faith, and after God's own heart, to have patiently followed Abram and his invisible God's promises to them all these years before her idea of Hagar.

Abram could have refused Sarai's advice to have a child through an Egyptian servant, just as he had been bold enough to refuse to heed the request of the King of Sodom to take the spoils of war to himself (Genesis 14:21-23). Abram believed he was already blessed, and that the blessing was the source of his prosperity, so he told the King of Sodom that he has vowed to God not to take nothing, not even a thread nor a sandal strap that belonged to another to add to his own possessions lest another could say he had made Abram rich. This is because when God told Abram, "I will bless you and you shall be a blessing," Abram understood that to mean that God would bless him first so that he could become a blessing. And when God blessed him he saw the immediate manifestation of this in his life. His servants could also see it such that the oldest servant of his house testified of how much God has greatly blessed him and indeed he has become great (Genesis 24:35). The men outside his household too attested to his blessing that he was revered among them as lord and a mighty prince (Genesis 23:6). Abram was indeed blessed and he was daily living in the consciousness of this fact because he could see how God's promises to give him inheritances came to pass, even so outside his homeland. By his consistent observation of how God had been dealing with him in the area of prosperity, Abram refused to be compromised in that area.

Abram had great faith in God's provision of this material blessing, and so he never failed any test in this respect; he trusted in God's promise to make him the father of blessing (Genesis 12:2-3). God had proved good on His promise to bless Abram outside his country, and so Abram could not be compromised in the area of material blessing.

So, then, why did Abram agree to Sarai's inimical request if he understood how the promise of his having children and becoming a father of nations would come to pass? Why did Abram not tell Sarah that what she wanted him to do was a wicked thing against her and God, just as Joseph told Potiphar's wife in Genesis 39:9? Or why did Abram not rebuke Sarai the way Job rebuked his wife and refused to take her advice to curse God (Job 2: 10)?

But Abram never even asked Sarai to consider what people would say—for instance that they lacked faith; that he would be committing adultery or no longer loved his wife because she could not bear him a child; that they would mock his God of inability to bring to pass His promises to Abram or that his descendants would be offspring of an Egyptian–a people whom God would prefer that they have no sexual dealings with. He made no attempt to do any of these things but went right in and slept with Hagar.

Could this suggest that Abram loved his wife so much not to let down her wishes and cravings? Or he had even been nursing this idea in his heart and Sarai just came to help him realize his longings to impregnate one of his slaves as an alternative to this delayed promise of having children? This was probably the case as evidenced by the fact that Abram made no protest. So what caused this man who was so blessed of God and so close to God as to be called "a friend of God" to abandon God's promise and go into a slave instead? The answer lies in *the blessing of Sarah*. Abram was not informed about the blessing of Sarah when all these things happened. He did not understand precisely how God would make him a father of nations as He had made him a father of blessing until God helped him to understand how he would do it. God sees the heart and thus could see in Abram's heart that he would continue to go in unto Sarai's handmaid, thereby further disrupting God's plan, and thus God quickly went to his rescue.

Before I proceed, let me explain that understanding 'how' a task can be done minimizes mistakes and similarly understanding how a promise will be fulfilled brings peace amidst storms that pose a threat to its fulfillment.

➢ God's instructions to Moses on how to rescue the children of Israel from the stronghold of Pharaoh created a resilience in Moses.

18

For instance, when he faced impossible challenges like convincing Pharaoh to let go of the Israelites, and the crossing the Red Sea with the Egyptian army's chariots about to descend upon them.

➢ Joshua felt his heart in his mouth when God passed the mantle of leadership of Israel to him at the death of Moses. Joshua relief came when God charged him to be strong and courageous rather than being faint-hearted. He got further consolation when He also said "No man shall be able to stand before you all the days of your life; and as I was with Moses so I will be with you, I will not leave you nor forsake you" (Joshua 1:5). At this point, I can perceive that the young man's fears and doubts were gradually melting away, however he still had worries unresolved by this words of assurance alone which God could read on his mind. Some of his worries included 'how' he would lead this multitude of rebellious and complaining people to the Promised Land. Thinking "Lord, ... what if along the way they want to go back to Egypt" and "Oh I'm not able to adequately cater for their needs as I do not have a rod to strike the rock to bring them water and to do many signs and miracles that could alleviate their sufferings" or "Lord, how will I know what to do when I am not like Moses who speaks to you face to face and to whom You gave guiding commandments to direct the affairs of these obstinate people?" God, listening to Joshua's thoughts, encouraged him of his ability to solve the problems of leadership. Assuring Joshua, He encouraged him to remain strong and courageous, not wavering at His promise. And as for his worries on what guidelines to follow in the absence of his face to face access to God, He told him, "look here Joshua, this book of the law shall not depart from your mouth, but you shall meditate on it day and night as you observe to do according to all that is written in it. Then your way shall be prosperous and shall you have good success" (Joshua 1:8). That is what he needed to be successful in his task. Therefore he stepped out in courage and began working towards the fulfillment of the assignment. In the process, he and his people were faced with the great Jordan River where God gave him clear instructions enabling him to lead Israel across the river. The next obstacle he confronted was entering into Jericho, a city whose walls were regarded as the most impregnable by width and tallest in height in all the world. The fall of the walls of Jericho after the Israelites obeyed His instruction, reinforced Joshua's faith in God's promise never to leave or forsake him. Joshua came to understand that the "How" was all he needed, whenever he had to accomplish a task ordered from above. Knowing what to do and when, helps to conserve resources in fulfilling the task.

➢ It was also mentioned that Jesus Himself knew what to do (John 6:6) whenever He was faced with challenges in the course of His assignment. When He was to depart from earth, He deeply understood the fact that His disciples would need to know and understand what they ought to do in their own course of fulfilling the assignment. So, giving them clear instructions He warned them not to start to carry out the assignment until they were endued from on high by the Holy Spirit (Act 1:4).

God is a loving father; He wants us to have understanding of His ways. He does not intend to leave us in the dark as there is no darkness in Him. That is why He came to Abram's rescue. Abram is indeed a father of faith as he rarely questioned God's orders to him. He took it head-on, without asking how it was to manifest.

*But just knowing God's plan for carrying out a task protects you from dealing with the wrong people or places.*

But just knowing God's plan for carrying out a task protects you from dealing with the wrong people or places. Abraham, who at the time of promise, had a vague understanding of the "how" for fulfillment of the blessing, got involved with the wrong person, Hagar. Meanwhile, Abraham's learned willingness to obey God's instruction were the seeds that bought about a change in his financial status. Knowing the 'how' in Abraham's case of having an heir in old age would have prevented the error of having an Ishmael. In this, I realized that the 'how' was already in the custody of Abraham but he did not have any clue about the promised heirs conception. I noticed from study, that God's dealings with Abraham were not with a rod like Moses or with a charge like Joshua, but with blessing. That's Abraham's hallmark—*the blessing* !!! Abraham perhaps thought that all God's promise of blessing to him only has to do with making him prosperous and becoming an exceedingly great nation. He understood the blessing for prosperity but had no understanding of what the blessing would do in bringing to life God's promise of an heir to him through his aged Sarah.

Hence, God helped Abram understand His ways of causing a woman who has not conceived to become fruitful. God wanted him to know and understand it, just as he understood how He was able to make a poor man like him become stupendously prosperous at retirement age, and even in a strange territory. So God told Abram how they do it in heaven to bring about on earth the promise to many of the fruit of the womb. God showed

Abram how he brings something out of nothing. At this point please follow me closely and ponder these secret because if you can fully grasp the mystery that is about to be unfolded, you will never lack any good thing in your life.

God said to Abram that in order for an elderly barren woman such as Sarai to conceive, He would have to bless her so that she would be able to bear him a son and become a mother of nations. *Yea, it is the blessing, sir!* It is the blessing that enables you to conceive and bear a child, no matter what the medical verdict is. Sarai case was both medically and physically impossible until God came to disclose how she would do the impossible (because with God all things are possible).

And God said to Abram, "As for Saria thy wife, thou shalt not call her name Sarai, but Sarah shall her name be. And I will bless her, and give thee a son also of her: yea, I will bless her, and she shalt be a mother of nations; kings of people shall be of her" (Genesis 17:15-16, KJV).

But why this repetition of blessing her, considering that God does not waste His words or play with words? What God is saying in laymen's terms in verse 16 is that, "As for Sarah thy wife, I (God) will bless her and she shall give birth to a son. Yea, I (God) will bless her indeed, and she shall become a mother of nations such that kings of people shall be from her." God was helping Abraham understand the process, so He said, "See, just as I changed your name from Abram (Man of Greatness) to Abraham (Father of Nations), I am changing your wife's name from Sarai (A Princess), to Sarah (A Queen). The same way I blessed you to become blessed with great prosperity is the same way I am going to bless Sarah to be a fertile one and bear you a son. And then in the way I blessed you indeed that you became a father of blessing: I will indeed bless Sarah to become the mother of nations, and by so doing my covenant with you (Abraham) in Genesis 17:4-6 will become a reality of your life." It was at this point that Sarai got included in His covenant to Abram of becoming exceedingly fruitful, by the blessing upon her as well. This was the point that God took the blessing of Abram to the next level by His blessing on Sarah. Abram blessings moved to the next cadre of blessing in the covenant through the impartation of Sarai's humanity to reproduce their kind. It is the blessing of Sarah that would translate him from being a husband to a father and Sarah too, from being a wife to a mother. In all these, He wanted to emphasize the knowledge of the working of the blessing.

In essence God was saying to Abraham, "I know you are an intelligent man and could interpret how my blessing works, even more so my blessing *indeed;* and I know in the same way when you put two and two together and work the equation in your mind, you will realize that it is the blessing that Sarah also needs, to bring forth a child." God was saying to him, "Do not forget that when I wanted you to be the richest man on earth, despite the fact that you moved out of your father's house in old age, and arrived in a strange land without really anything, I simply engaged the blessing for you to become so rich. Thus, in the same manner, I will engage the blessing for Sarah thy wife so that she will bear you a son. "We need to remember that to God the blessing implies 'an impartation for result, that is, the transference of strength, ability, and power to become what he intended'. It was not normal for an old man to leave his country without a penny for another land, and there became a possessor of great and innumerable assets. Nothing explains that transformation more than the blessing! In the same way, Sarah, an old woman who had passed the age of menopause and no longer delights in sexual activities could conceive only by an invocation imploring the divine fertilizing power.

Then Abraham understood the secret—that it was the blessing *indeed,* likewise upon Sarah that would make her become a mother of nations and him a father of nations. He now fully comprehended all that God had been promising him all those years about having children. Because Abraham understood the language of the blessing, he never doubted it again. Abraham believed that as the blessing working upon him had ended his own years of financial struggle, in the same way, it was the blessing working upon Sarah that would end her years of waiting. So we see that once Abraham received the secret of the blessing, he had the strength, informed by knowledge, to wait another one year for the promise to come to pass (Genesis 21:5). God could have possibly brought the promise to pass within that one year interval without precisely revealing to Abraham how He intended to do it. But being God, He already knew there would be a time, when through this mystery, the waiting seeds of Abraham would become blessed with their own long awaited children.

When God spoke to him about how He would bring it to pass by pronouncing the blessing upon Sarah, Abraham was 99 years old. When Sarah bore Isaac, Abraham was 100 years old! He waited for the promise this time because he understood how God would do it. And that is why Abraham did not laugh, nor argue with the three 'men' who paid him a courtesy visit in Genesis 18. Abraham understood that it was the blessing that would make the good news they delivered to him and Sarah come to pass. But Sarah laughed at the same news! Why? This is because it was Abraham to whom God had been speaking concerning bearing a child, and the covenant of making him an exceedingly great nation. And it was Abraham who had tasted the working of the blessing and had come to understand what the blessing could do. God had explained it to him in a language he already understood, and for that one year he was calm and at peace about the fact that he would become a father.

Sarah laughed, however, because she was not informed about the working of the blessing. That is why the men spoke in a language that Sarah could understand when they said, "Is there anything too hard for the Lord? That at the time appointed Sarah shall have a son" (Genesis 18:14). She understood that clearly, but Abraham understood much more the blessing of Sarah and for this reason Abraham passed God's second test—sacrificing Isaac. Abraham realized that if he sacrificed Isaac, the blessing could give him another even if his time left on earth was short. He passed the test this time! He did not even question God when God told him to go and sacrifice Isaac, his only son whom he loves so much. We need to remember that this is the same Abraham who had bargained with God and pressed the buttons of mercy for the righteous not to be destroyed with the wicked when God told him He would destroy all the people of Sodom and Gomorrah (Genesis 18:20-33).

The same Abraham who had put God on hold for the

righteous souls in Sodom could also have thrown a challenge at God in regard to his son of promise. He might have contended with God that God was contradicting himself by giving him such a dreadful command given all that has transpired on the journey of Abraham and Sarah thus far in getting a child. Given all that, how could God make such a demand? He could also have reminded God that killing Isaac would put him and Sarah back to square one–barren as before. He could have pleaded for compassion– citing how substantially more agonizing it would be for them to see the long-awaited child pass away, even as their own future was fading.

So are you not also surprised to find that Abraham was not interested in bargaining with God this time, as he was placing his only righteous son Isaac on the altar? So why did he not do it? Here's why: He had come to understand the blessing of Sarah.

God put Abraham to this test to examine his depth of understanding of the blessing of Sarah that He taught him. Remember that this test of Abraham came unannounced. God never told him beforehand that "your first seed that I promised you shall you slay." We all know that teachers assess their students' understanding  of the course material by giving a test whose questions are not known beforehand. In this way, they are able to assess which students understand all that has been taught in the course. That was exactly the drama that unfolded here between God and Abraham in Genesis 22. God just wanted to put to the test Abraham's understanding of the blessing of Sarah, so that Abraham would understand the extent to which his understanding of the promised blessing had developed. *And see what happened!* Abraham did not prove otherwise. He passed the test. He proved to God that he could never fail that test again as he had failed the first time out of ignorance of the workings of the blessing of Sarah.

It was at this point that Abraham did not stagger at the promises of God regarding him and Sarah's conception of children. He had been given adequate information and revelation of the blessing of Sarah which will make the promise of an heir to him a reality. Being fully convinced now after a detailed explanation of the blessing of Sarah; he did not waver at the promise of God concerning conception understanding that He who has promised is able to perform it too in this case.

I submit to you, at this point that it is the blessing of Sarah working in you that will enable you to conceive and bear your own baby! The blessing of Sarah is the cure for the curses of barrenness. The very word "blessing" means *empowered to become*. Abraham was empowered to become prosperous and wealthy but Sarah had not been empowered to become a mother. The blessing of Sarah was the "empowerment to conceive or the empowerment to become pregnant". God changed the name of Abram to Abraham because he had cut a covenant of blessing with him and then also changed the name of Sarai to Sarah because the covenant of blessing to become pregnant had been pronounced, and once the blessing is pronounced the working power in the blessing runs swiftly to change the status of the blessed.

Note that this was the same thing that happened to Jacob when God first changed his name and blessed him (Genesis 32:28-29). Whenever the blessing is released everything changes. An aged body changes and becomes strong enough to carry a baby when the blessing is working. This empowerment to conceive is tailored to the gender with a womb, which is why the blessing was not pronounced on Abraham, a man (and thus without a womb). It takes a woman to harness this blessing of empowerment to become pregnant. This blessing is peculiar to women but men, too, need to be informed about it so they can harness it on behalf of their wives. God will not pronounce this blessing on men lest He reverse His work of creation, since it was His handiwork to make only women conceive and bear children. So it is exclusively reserved for women.

# Scriptural Notes

- Genesis 1:1-22

- Genesis 11:30

- Genesis 12: 2-3

- Genesis 14: 21-23

- Genesis 16:6

- Genesis 17: 4-6

- Genesis 17: 15-16

- Genesis.18: 14, 20-33

- Genesis 21: 5

- Genesis 23: 6

- Genesis 24: 35

- Genesis 30: 1

- Genesis 32: 28-29

- Genesis 39: 9

- Joshua 1: 5, 8

- 1 Samuel 1:8

- Job 2:10

- John 6:6

- Act 1: 4

# CHAPTER THREE

*The Blessing of Sarah is Located in the Spirit*

*And I bless her, and give you a son from her! Yea, I will bless her, and she shall*

*become a mother of nations; kings of people shall be from her*

*- Genesis 17:16p*

---

**The Blessing of Sarah is the blessing of the Womb**

In chapter two, we took a close look at the blessing of Sarah, which we can summarize in these terms: "The blessing of Sarah is the blessing of the Womb." In Genesis 27 it is apparent how Isaac, Abraham's son prioritises the need for the blessing before his demise. Abraham's grandson, Jacob, also understood the importance of the blessing of Sarah (Genesis 49:25) that Abraham could not initially comprehend. Before his death, he blessed each of his twelve sons and at Joseph's turn; he changed the order to that of the blessings of the breast

31

and of the womb. This was because the promise to Abraham, Isaac, and Jacob that their seeds shall become a multitude of people to evolve into a great nation was to materialize through Joseph. The manifestation of the Abrahamic blessing was to commence from Joseph. In Genesis 46, God spoke to Jacob that he should not be afraid to go to Egypt where Joseph lives, for He would make him there a great nation. Meanwhile, prior to his departure, God had made Joseph, his son, become a ruler throughout all the land of Egypt.

Since the days of Abraham, none of his seeds had become a multitude of people, and there was less talk of growing in number unto nationhood until Joseph came on the scene who shall push the people to the ends of the earth (Deuteronomy 33:16-17). Isaac a seed of Abraham was one person. Isaac's seeds, Esau and Jacob were two persons although God referred to them as two nations. Jacob's twelve children put together either could not make a nation, yet the promise was to become a multitude of people, a great nation that will inherit a new land through which all the earth would be blessed. However, the presence of Joseph in Egypt would contribute to bringing the promise of becoming a multiple of people into fruition. They were to grow and multiply into a multitude enough to form a nation first in Egypt. This was the insight Jacob had, that prompted him to first of all release the blessing on Joseph and his two sons (Ephraim and Manasseh) to grow into a multitude of people according to Genesis 48: 15-16. While he blessed the lads, he also established that his name be named upon them as part of the making of this great nation arising from Egypt. This was how they were named after Israel (formerly Jacob) and are referred to even today as the children of Israel.

Despite that Jacob had already pronounced this blessing upon Joseph and his sons, he repeatedly pronounced same blessing upon Joseph when he was blessing all his sons in Genesis 49. Let me pause here to explain that the Abraham blessing of becoming a great nation is futuristic. When God blessed Abraham, what God delivered to him was the future. Abraham saw the days of Joseph, Jesus, and my days. Abraham also saw your days as well as those of your children and did believe and rejoiced that what he saw would come to pass. This was what Jesus described in John 8:56 as "Abraham saw my days and rejoiced." Abraham saw the things which were not as though they were and notice God calling them forth as though they were (Romans 4: 17). In the same vein, Isaac blessed his seeds concerning things to come (Hebrews 11:20) being pre-informed of the promise of God to make of them a great nation. Therefore, he pronounced them blessed with the blessings of Abraham which is God giving them of the dew of heaven and the fatness of the earth (Genesis 27:28) that he witnessed in his father Abraham.

> *When God blessed Abraham, what God delivered to him was the future*

Jacob on the contrary had an insight into the fullness of blessing that would make his seeds become a multitude of people to form the great nation. He had a foresight into what the combination of the blessing of Abraham and of Sarah could do in the materialization of this great nation promised to him and his fathers. Moreover, he knew what he had seen after God spoke with him (Genesis 46:3) about the offspring of promise becoming a great nation through Joseph's presence in Egypt and as a result he reiterated the same blessing, expounding on it this time. Therefore, Jacob blessed Joseph, the fruitful bough, with the blessing of the breast and of the womb so that nothing can stop their growing into a throng of people in Egypt and subsequently. He actually pronounced both the blessing of Abraham and the blessing of Sarah (Genesis 49:25). These two blessings are comprised of a fourfold blessing (of heavens, of earth, of breast, and of womb) which makes up the fullness of blessing. That is to Joseph he said "would be blessed with the blessings of heaven above and with the blessing of the deep that lies beneath (which is the blessing of Abraham) and with blessing of the breasts and of the womb (which is the blessing of Sarah)" so that no affliction, curse, or inimical decree could prevent them from growing in number as God promised their fathers. These two blessings worked so much in them that they grew mightily in Egypt, outnumbered the Egyptians, and they never lacked provisions too (Exodus 1:7). This scripture depicts the outcome of the workings of the blessing upon them—they grew exceedingly mighty such that the land of Egypt was filled with them.

Considering also that God told Jacob that He would not leave him until He had done everything that He had spoken to him (Genesis 28), Jacob did not only have this experience but also saw the first king of that royal line (Joseph) coming out of his offspring. Even though it was to Abraham that God told about having kings of people coming from them, Jacob, a seed of Abraham, saw the first king of promise. Isaac, Abraham's son was not a king, so Abraham did not witness the manifestation of this blessing of coming kings in his life time neither did any king arose from Isaac's off spring. It was from Jacob's and that is why he could say in Genesis 49:26 that his own blessings have exceeded the blessing of his ancestors, Abraham and Isaac. Aside that he saw the first king of that royal line from his offspring, he also witnessed in his lifetime, an emerging increase in the number of people from that lineage which gives him the assurance that the promise to him and his fathers of becoming a great nation would be fulfilled without fail. What's more! He also saw that the King of kings and the everlasting One, Jesus Christ, was going to come out of this great nation. For this reason, he mentioned in the same verse that "his own blessings have prevailed above that of his progenitors even unto the everlasting hills". Jesus is a manifestation of the Abrahamic blessing but the commencement for its manifestation was centred on Joseph, the fruitful bough.

*The blessing of Sarah working on their lives was too strong for the afflictions hurled*

Jacob had seventy people came with him into Egypt (Genesis 46:27) but numerous people went out of Egypt because the blessing of the womb was their fertility pills. That is why the decree of a king Pharaoh who did not know Joseph could not delay their conception or delivery. The more the children of Israel were subjected to hard labour, the more they grew in size and the more they were afflicted; the more they multiplied (Exodus 1:12) in Egypt. It was such an unprecedented occurrence that rather than the children of Israel being afraid of Pharaoh's decree of torture and for the destruction of the seeds of their wombs; the Egyptians were living in dread of them. The blessing of Sarah working on their lives was too strong for the afflictions hurled at them. Not even decrees were potent enough to hold back their women from conceiving and putting to bed. It vividly demonstrates how the workings of the blessings of the breast and of the womb could ward off barrenness and aids a small number of people to become a multitude. Not one of their women was barren nor were any of their men impotent... because the blessing was working. Even the midwives attested to the working of the blessing upon their woman—proclaiming that this breed of women is exceptional, because they gave birth before they even arrive! What an unstoppable blessing was at work!

More so, after they had left Egypt, their women were still conceiving and giving birth through the wilderness journeys. Pregnancy, for them, was not a disease. Despite the absence of good living conditions and medical supplies like bed, pampers, sanitary towels, feeding bottles, the women had safe deliveries, weaning the new born babes with just breast milk. In fact, the decades of their residing in the wilderness could not prevent the Israelites from conceiving and giving birth to children. One would have thought that living in a wilderness for forty (40) years without proper balanced diets at their reach would affect their fertility, but it did not! Their women were conceiving and putting to birth while in the wilderness where they fed mostly on manna (a food with a high concentrate of carbohydrate). It's a fact in the medical world that balanced diets are compulsory meals for potency and fertility in people all over the world. The Israelites in the wilderness finding their way from Egypt were an exception, as they proved the cycle wrong. Despite their consumption of manna consistently for 40 years, Joshua recorded in his memoirs that male and female children were born on their way (Joshua 5:5). Remarkable, huh!

Subsequently, even at a time when they were scattered in various countries due to their disobedience, He gathered the remnant of the Israelites out of all these countries and declared that they shall yet become fruitful and increase into a nation as they were (Jeremiah 23:3). He did not leave the famished and exploited remnant without the blessing to replenish. In fact, while in the land of captivity, the Lord charged them to marry wives and give birth to sons and daughters; and that their sons and daughters be given in marriage that they may bear sons and daughters and increase there without diminishing (Jeremiah 29:6). In this charge of the Lord to them is an accompanied blessing to conceive and increase greatly while on hostage in the land of captivity.

*Securing the blessing is more important than the focus on the limitations to bearing and the search for alternatives*

If these women who did not have a tenth in quality of the living conditions available today, could bear and deliver healthy children, then we are in a better position for fertility. Besides, if these women, who did not know Jesus and had never partaken of His blood and flesh, could not be prevented from conceiving, then you are in a better covenant towards fruitfulness. More than just food was working in the children of Israel. The men of Israel had healthy sperm count to fertilize a baby in the absence of balanced diet, medical facilities and gynecologist's advice. All they had was the blessing! I tell you that the man in your life has the best opportunity today more than the men of Israel and with the blessing also at work in you; you are in for a same experience of fruitfulness. From these examples, securing the blessing is more important than the focus on the limitations to bearing and the search for alternatives.

A lot has been explicitly revealed from the scriptures to help you fully understand the blessing of Sarah, and now I would like to show you how you can connect with this blessing and harness it in your own life.

## IN THE SPIRIT NOT IN THE BODY

First, we must understand that the blessing of Sarah has its origin in a work of the Spirit. It is therefore located in the spirit and not in the body. It is not a medical issue but a spiritual one. In this case, the Spirit aids that part or bit of humanity unto gestation and normal birth. To help you further comprehend this mystery, let me start by using the example of the blessing of Abraham. Abraham left his father, Terah's house, without anything and went to a foreign land where he knew no one. He was in a strange land with no family to support him while he got his bearings. But before long, we find that he has become a land owner with cattle and great possessions. This poor man had become very rich and most likely was the wealthiest man of his time. This is not a typical human experience. Realistically, we would expect him to suffer financial hardship since he went to a foreign land with little or no money. But he not only survived but *thrived*: kings reckoned with him because of his wealth. Even the Philistines envied his son Isaac who had inherited all his possessions.

This only happens when a blessing is at work in a person's life. The blessing had been pronounced upon Abraham's humanity and that magnetises riches and favours to him in strange lands. He has been aided by the invisible to become blessed and a blessing to many. The blessing at work in his life rendered him immune to the curses of poverty and hardship prevailing over other men of his times. Notice that this immunity to the curse of hardship was coupled with the fact that Abraham was faithful in his tithing and did not add other people's belongings to his own. Thus, the working of the blessing could not be truncated.

In our day, I have heard some preachers tell stories of how they were led into a city for the work of the ministry and entered the place with little or no money but received blessing and today own properties not only in those cities but in those countries. My own life is an example. I come from a humble, so-called "poor" background; I should not be where I am today because my parents could not afford to give me much. The blessing was at work as I went through my undergraduate program in a university where fees and the cost of living were quite expensive without a bank loan. After completing my studies, I was able to get a job without the help of any man in a place where ordinarily people of my calibre (i.e., from a poor background) do not easily get in. *How?* It was the working of the blessing.

My parents could not afford to pay my way for an internationally-recognized professional examination to become a chartered accountant because examination fees are due in 'hard' currency. But I was conscious of the working of the blessing upon my life, so I took a giant step to enrol knowing full well that my parents or family members could not afford it. I paid for the exams by the workings of the blessing of Abraham upon my life! I wrote the stages and, by the workings of the blessing, today, I am a Certified Chartered Accountant. What is more, my parents, who could not have afforded to send me abroad to study for my postgraduate qualification, are blessed today to see their daughter sponsored to undertake her Master's program in one of the top schools in the United Kingdom, with tuition and all living expenses paid for by the government because the blessing is working.

My parents' life savings could not have been able to fetch all these for me but the blessing did. There are yet many other blessing that I am not able to disclose in this book that I have enjoyed through the consciousness of the working of the blessing of Abraham upon my life. It is much better than decades of labour, and it is real. It actually works and I attest to you that it is still working to this very day. That is the same way the blessing of Sarah also works for those who can access it and understand its workings enough to engage it to become mothers of children.

It is interesting to know and see from Job 1:10 how that even Satan attested to the working of the blessing as tantamount to increment in substance. Satan, our arch enemy, understands the mystery of the blessing so well that he accused God of putting a barrier on his operations by His blessing on Job.

Verse .10: "Hast not thou made an hedge about him, and about his house, and about all that he hath on every side? Thou hast blessed the work of his hands, and his substance is increased in the land".

He bears this out to God concerning Job that His blessing upon him has made his substance increased greatly in the land just as it was with father Abraham. I believe that in the same manner,

Satan also does affirm to the working of the blessing of the breast and of the womb as resulting into increment in the fruit of the body on earth. He understands the power of the blessing and what the blessing is capable of doing in men and women's lives. As the blessing upon a man culminates into increase in his greatness and substance; so also does the blessing upon a woman culminates into increment in the fruit of her womb. The blessing is real and its workings on the life of a man or woman can turn the course of their life around.

This blessing of Sarah can only be found in the supernatural realm–the realm of the Spirit. It is wrought by the breaths and workings of the Holy Spirit through Christ Jesus. The blessing is by the Spirit–and not by the sperm–to see to it that you are blessed to have your own children. It is by the Spirit and not by the state of your woman for her to carry a baby in her womb. It is the reception of an operation of the Spirit on our own humanity to conceive. When it is the Spirit working, the natural fact that you have passed the age of menopause is irrelevant. Why? This is because the Spirit rejuvenates! When the Spirit of God is working the blessings on you, there can be no barrier in your womb to your having a Seed come out from your body. Why? It is because the Spirit recreates and as well exterminate. The Spirit cannot be blocked from working the blessing on you at His initiation. This was the case of Sarah! God released His working Spirit of blessings on Sarah such that even in old age Sarah received strength to conceive. That is, she received the empowerment to become pregnant through the working of the Spirit.

For this reason it was said, that from a man as good as dead and a woman as good as dead were born children as numerous as the stars of the sky (Hebrews 11:11-12). That bit of their humanity responsible for childbirth was worn out and packed up. It had been certified non-functional and immaterial for conception. Sarah was likened to a dead woman at the age she gave birth to Isaac. This shows that her state was indeed hopeless to have her body compared with those whose dwelling is in graves. At the advent of the blessing, however, she did not only give birth to Isaac but her dried and deadened breast recuperated that she had enough breast milk to wean the child unto maturity since no baby food existed in those days. In our contemporary world, it is absolutely impossible for a 90-year-old woman to become pregnant, much less to have the wherewithal to deliver the baby. When it is the blessing working by the Spirit, however, a 120-year-old woman with a year to live can conceive and also be given strength to deliver the baby. Today, even at 80 some women are already bent over with osteoporosis and are no longer physically able to hold a baby in their womb protectively for nine months, but it happened with Sarah because the blessing was at work on her life. She could not be denied by natural phenomena.

The Spirit of God imparted her humanity and further enabled her to receive supernatural strength to push out the baby at that advanced age. The baby did not die in her womb because the blessing was working upon her, so she made it after all. The Spirit also worked out the blessing of the breast upon Sarah for her to become a woman with a milky breast to breastfeed the baby to maturity. The same thing happened to Elizabeth, who gave birth to John the Baptist in her old age. That is why God allowed an angel who had been standing in the presence of God since creation and thus had seen how God performs His working of the blessing of the womb to take the message to Zechariah the father of John and to Mary the mother of Jesus (Luke 1:19, 26-37). This was to enable us understand how the blessing of the womb is carried out in heaven.

By virtue of his position as one constantly standing in the presence of God awaiting His next instruction, Angel Gabriel had been seeing God working this blessing upon Sarah, Rebecca, Rachel, Hannah, and many other women of old who were once called barren.

He came from heaven to explain to Mary the working of the blessing of Sarah. The angel first of all greeted Mary with the words "rejoice highly favoured one, blessed are you among women" (Luke1:28). And the Bible says that Mary was wondering about this greeting. For him to say she was blessed among women means that there were some women who were not blessed with the blessing that Mary was about to experience. In other words the angel was saying to Mary, "Mary, by the virtue of my office in the presence of God, where I have been seeing my Master do things for thousands of years now, and by my close and regular observation of what He does and how He has been doing it in heaven to see that some women conceive on earth, I have seen it from the way the Master has done it for you again that it is your turn for the blessing, and that is why I could not but greet you as the blessed one among other women. *Yea, you have been blessed!* " This was the same greeting that Elizabeth lauded at the arrival of Mary in her house. Elizabeth speaking out with a loud voice by the moving of the Holy Spirit confirms the words of the angel that

Mary was blessed indeed among women (Luke1:41-42) for her conception to take place.

Before I go further, it would be appropriate to clarify here that this description does not in any way down play the uniqueness of the birth of Jesus Christ. He was a 'holy one', whose conception needed to be purified by an absence of sexual activities and untainted by sperm. It was a conception actually resulting from a romance between divinity and humanity. Therefore, He was conceived of the Holy Spirit. In this sense, the birth of Jesus is exclusive though the process of His birth expresses to us the possibilities that exist in a work of the Spirit which is also available to us to avail.

The angel then proceeded to deliver the message to Mary of what he meant by calling her "blessed among women," that she would conceive in her womb and bring forth a son. At that, Mary became more afraid and confused, wondering how that could be real, knowing full well that she was a virgin and had known no sperm. And right here the angel gave the blast! "Mary, it is the working of the Spirit of the Holy God upon you that will make it become real. Yea, the empowerment to become pregnant that comes from the Highest will overshadow you that you will not only become pregnant but you will give birth to the baby". To top it off, the angel said to her, "look at your relative Elizabeth who was called barren but has also conceived in her old age, for with God nothing shall be impossible by the working of the empowerment to become pregnant" (paraphrase of Luke 1:36-37).

I must submit to you here that this is the blessing of Sarah of the Old Testament repeated in the life of Elizabeth in the New

Testament for us to become inspired and harness this secret in our own age and time. As Sarah was blessed in her old age to conceive a son, so also was Elizabeth blessed to conceive a son in old age. Blessed are those who believe the saying, for they shall experience the performance of the working of the blessing of womb. This is because with the working of the Spirit of the blessing of the womb, the donation of sperm might not be a necessary factor and the agedness of the body irrelevant for conception. Do not forget that Abraham's body was also considered as good as dead, his sperms not an exception, because they were already seen as incapable for fertilization, yet he was aided when the Lord visited. *It was not more of the sperm that did it, sir!* This was more than sperm could do. It was the Spirit of the Lord aiding them to become enabled to conceive without fleshly contribution. Is not this God wonderful!

The blessing of Sarah is a work of the Spirit and hence is a part of the ministry of the Holy Spirit and a demonstration of God's power. I said earlier in a previous paragraph, that the process of Jesus' birth discloses to us the possibilities that exist in a work of the Spirit. This statement is the truth! This is because there are many description of the activities of the Holy Spirit in the Bible that demonstrate to us the world of possibilities that exist in the workings of the Spirit and available to us if only we could harness them. Usually, these are underlying statements or illustrations that make obvious God's original intension, design plans or Kingdom practice; because really in the beginning some things were not so intended. A good example is from the saying of Jesus who existed since the beginning that "It is the Spirit who gives life; the flesh profits nothing" going by John 6:63. This is to tell us that a living thing can only culminate from the work of the Spirit. That is why the apostle John affirms that all things were through Him and without His contribution was nothing made (John 1:3). This is a dramatic expression of the reality of their operations in Heaven.

Furthermore, the narrative of Paul to the Romans in chapter 8:2 goes on to make clear that there is a law of the Spirit of life that makes free in Christ Jesus. Paul is aware of the existence of a law of the Spirit of life that set free from every other law whether sin, curses, or death. This realistic illustration of Paul of a work of the Spirit connotes that there would be a law of the Spirit of blessing that exterminates all unwanted plantings that was not so in the beginning. Life and blessings are the work of the Spirit while the law of curses and death is under the three fold ministry of Satan, that is, to 'kill', 'steal' and 'destroy'. Hence, for every law of curses is a corresponding law from the Spirit to nullify it. So from history of God's creation, the law of the Spirit of blessing makes free from all laws of curses of whatever kind.

The same way the law of the Spirit of life sets free from the law of sin and death is in same manner, the law of the Spirit of blessing of the womb sets free from the law of curses of barrenness. This is the reason Paul was admonishing that they should live by the Spirit and not by the flesh. Fleshly activities in marriage is good and does not in any way defile the marriage bed, however, a production of fruits from your flesh is more than just sperm could do. We could see this expressly in the case of Elkanah and Hannah, who despite engaging in sexual intercourse could still not conceive until the Lord stepped in (I Samuel 1:19b). That it is by the working of the Spirit of the blessing of the womb is an extraordinary phenomenon but this has been the precedence in the Kingdom. This method is what God repeatedly demonstrated at creation and more so when He wanted His own chosen ones to increase in number. It was the Spirit giving them a great impetus towards fruitfulness in their flesh.

This way of God bringing about fruitfulness has an element of revelation about its workings. It is an awareness of a Spiritual truth on the efficacy of pronouncement of the blessing. The pronouncement of the blessing upon is the most powerful arching measure over curses, and the tongue is a very powerful gift in the pronouncement of blessings of whatever kind. God taught us this in His work of creation and the seeds of Abraham too, from Scriptures, showed us many examples of the significance of pronouncement of blessings. The growth and intense awareness of God's method towards conception of the body will without delay enable you to contact the blessings of the womb. It would be a rewarding experience for young women to grow up opened to the reality of this truth of God's way to conception. This truth is to make us grow in wisdom that your long awaited blessing would come to earth after the order of His work in the Spirit. Real life examples and testimonies of people in our own time have been documented in the last chapter of this book to brace up your faith.

## HOPE FOR YOU!

If only you can yet hope once more, you would be glad you did!

I like a piece of Naomi's story that relate to the blessing of the breast and of the womb. According to her life's story in Ruth chapter 1; she knew if only she could hope once more, she could yet have a husband and bear sons at her old age. She saw the possibility that existed in hoping against hope even as she repeated to her two daughters-in-law to return from following her since she no longer have sons to marry them. Although she acknowledged that she is too old to have sons left in her womb for them to marry, she still saw that with hope, it was not an impossible occurrence (Ruth1:12). Naomi, a woman who understands and could interpret God's dealings with her in her own days, described hope in God as a key to obtaining a husband at old age and the strength to conceive sons. This connotes that no matter how old you are; everything is possible with God if you can hope in Him. Naomi, an aged woman, could see possibilities in her seemingly hopeless case by hoping in God. With hope, her fears was not that she may not get a man to marry her or that she may not conceive sons at her old age, but with the fact that the ladies might not be able to wait for the babies to grow up into men. If Naomi could still envisage a comeback and could see a wealth of possibilities in her hopeless case; then you can also see the possibilities embedded in your impossibilities when you hope in the Spirit that gives life.

Dear, I see hope for you in the working of the Spirit of the Highest. Your case is not too hard for Him to handle. He only wants you to understand the working of the blessing of the womb so you can engage your faith through the working of the Spirit to receive your sons and daughters. You are nearer there now than ever! You are on the verge of bringing forth by the release of the blessing of Sarah in you, working mightily in you and in your spouse to bring you to the conception that you have long waited for. You can become part of those who will bring forth children after the working of the Spirit and not just after the working of the flesh.

Many children are born into the world today after the working of the flesh and are not well-cared for nor brought up in the way of the Lord. Many young people out there in the world mess around and become pregnant after the working of the flesh, so how much more will you, who are of more knowledge than they, receive the blessing of a baby when you engage the working of the blessing. Shall you not become pregnant after the working of the Spirit upon you? Can you imagine your coming out of a romance with the Holy Spirit and not becoming pregnant instantaneously after the working of the Spirit? Would it be impossible for God to impregnate you after the work of the Spirit with Him? No way, that dead womb will pop open! And that shut womb shall have its gate continually opened! It cannot resist the working of the Spirit of God because the working of the Spirit is superior to the working of the flesh. The Spirit of God cannot be stopped when it determines to work the blessing of Sarah upon anyone.

It penetrates through without any obstruction and gets your ovaries filled with His living Spirit to form a baby in your womb. Remember how in the beginning, when God created the first man, he formed an adult using the dust. I mean, God formed a full-grown man and not a baby boy who was formed in the beginning when the first man was created. First, this tells us that God could manufacture an adult if He so desired and not a baby who will take years to mature into an adult. Can you imagine the might and power of that God? Can not a God who did not form a 'baby' Adam at first and allow him to grow up over time but formed him straightaway into an 'adult' being, much more form a baby inside of you? Of course He can!

For us to understand His works properly, He repeated that act again when he took a rib from Adam to form Eve into a full-grown female and not into a baby girl, just for us to be convinced about His abilities to create children for us. Another insight here is that when God wanted to create the woman, He did not use the sperm of man but used His rib to signify to us that He does things as it pleases Him because He is God. He knew that in the future medical doctors would tell some couples that they could not conceive a child because the man has a low sperm count, and so He did this to show us that it is possible even without the contribution of sperm.

This ability to create adults straight off without making them first babies was what was on God's mind when He told Noah He was going to wipe out all living beings on the face of the earth. Noah would probably be calculating, like any of us today, how God would get people to start afresh on the earth. Would it not take a long time for the earth to be occupied again even if God created another man and woman? Would it not take years for them to mature and start to procreate? How would God do it to have the human beings replaced? All these are the thoughts of man, but God knows that He could create adults who would not need to first of all grow from babyhood to adulthood to start the creation all over again. He could do this way. That is why He could think of wiping all men from the face of the earth in the first place (Genesis 6:7). If it were going to cost Him to create fresh human beings the idea of wiping out all men from the planet earth would not have crossed His mind in the first instance. He must have counted the costs, and He could see His Spirit hovering over the face of the deep again and creating fresh adults who will fulfill His planned agenda for the earth.

Furthermore, after God formed the first man in Genesis 2:7, man did not become a living being until He breathed into his nostrils. This is to show us that it is the Spirit of God that makes man and not so much the working of the sperm in the woman. David attested to this when he wrote about how God created man, saying that He commanded and they were created (Psalm 148:5). In other words, human beings cannot be born unless the Father has commanded it by the working of His Spirit. Why am I saying all these? To help you channel your energies in the right direction. Rather than thinking that your husband is the problem, or that your wife is the problem, use that energy to think of how "the problem" lies in the fact that you have not yet engaged the working of the Spirit of the blessing of Sarah and then settle down with God whose Spirit gives life and can impregnate the woman.

Redirect all of the energy and effort you have expended seeking one doctor after another and spending exorbitant sums of money on so-called "wonder drugs" and undergoing all kinds of tests to simply sit down with the Word of the Spirit that can give life. Enough of the weight of swallowing drugs and undergoing endless tests! It is not a sin to do so; however, it is a weight that can be laid aside when we embrace His wisdom on these issues. Do not allow all of these to shift your focus from Him since there is a tendency to get preoccupied with these exercises and ultimately ceases to look to Him. Jesus has put in clear terms for us that it is the Spirit who gives life; the flesh profits nothing. The medicine you need is the Spirit who gives life and can work out the blessing of the womb on your life to conceive your own children. You have gone around searching for alternatives when the way to become pregnant is simply in the Spirit, so why not locate it there?

Engage the word of God and the ministry of the empowerment of the Holy Spirit to harness the blessing of Sarah, which is the blessing of the womb, to enable you to carry your own children. I have heard a woman testify that her womb was removed during an operation some years ago but that today she has given birth to a bouncing baby boy after she sat down to engage the Spirit that gives life. Her testimony is fully shared in the last chapter of this book. The sexual activities married couples engage in are good but that is not what really gives life. You have tried that all these years and have not conceived your own promised children, so why not try to harness the blessing of Sarah that comes through the empowerment of the Spirit of the Highest so you can testify as well?

If you will harness all these scriptural truth portraying the workings of blessing of the womb there is no way that you will not become pregnant. The knowledge of the Word of God is your most powerful force within. With it, you will reproduce life within you. Hear what God says again to you on this matter in Isaiah 54:5. God is reminding all the women who have been bothered about the fact that their husband is reported to have a low sperm count that they should not worry because He (Spirit of God and the power of conception) will become their husband just to see them conceive. In short, God reiterated, "perhaps you still doubt the first statement that I, your Maker, will be your Husband, but see, I am even the Lord of Hosts and that is my name." In other words, God is saying, "I have got hosts of sperm in my custody that you need not worry about the fact that your earthly husband has low sperm count. I am your husband with a 'host' of sperm count to help boost your faith and not only that but with a 'host' of ways to impregnate you even if you do not have a womb!"

## GOD IS GREAT, IS HE NOT?

That is why He said you should spread out your tents and makes more chairs for your dining table because very soon your twins, triplets, and children shall surround your table, so start living in the consciousness of the working of the blessing of Sarah on your life and never again doubt it that you shall soon become a mother.

God respects our faith and is pleased by it. There is no faith in negative confession or entertaining negative thoughts. There is no faith in quarrelling with your husband or wife because you think he or she is the problem and vice versa. There is no faith in flitting about from one doctor to another and spending a lot of money on drugs and endless tests and operations without any commensurate result. Why not connect with the Spirit of the blessing of Sarah? When I was a teenager in secondary school, a doctor once told my parents that I was asthmatic and that, if left untreated, it could take my life. I knew something was wrong with my breathing but did not know it was asthma until the doctor's test showed it. Although I was young then, I still remember the teachings of my pastor that emphasize that it is not of God to be sick or to have sicknesses in our bodies, and I could remember since that day we received the doctor's report my parents started to live in fear for me. My dad spent his meager salary buying me different types of inhalers to always take with me to school and wherever I might go. But before long I got fed up and then in my own little understanding knelt down and prayed to this God whom my pastor spoke so much about who could heal me of asthma and instantly He did.

Since then till now, I have had no further symptoms of asthma for these 12 years, and since then I have been walking in the consciousness of the blessing of divine health and that is why my parents have had no reason to take me to the hospital again. It can happen for you, too, if you believe in the Father of the Spirit of all flesh who desires that we become blessed with all spiritual blessing, and can empower you to become a parent. He can and He will do it for you. I see you getting pregnant by the working of His Spirit of the blessing of the womb upon your life in Jesus name. Believe the word of God and not the word of your doctor and you shall experience miracle childbirth through the moving of the Spirit!

# Scriptural Notes

- Genesis 2: 7

- Genesis 6: 7

- Genesis 27: 1-28

- Genesis 28: 3-4; 12-15

- Genesis 46: 2-4, 27

- Genesis 48: 15-16

- Genesis 49: 25-26

- Exodus 1: 12

- Exodus 1:7, 12

- Deuteronomy 33: 16-17

- Joshua 5: 5

- Ruth 1: 12

- I Samuel 1:19b

- Psalm 148: 5

- Isaiah 54: 5

- Jeremiah 23: 3; 29: 6

- Luke 1: 19,26-37,41-42

- John 1:3; 6:63; 8:56

- Romans 4: 17; 8:2

- Hebrews 11: 11-12, 20

# CHAPTER FOUR

*In the Beginning even "Mother Earth" was Barren*

*And I will bless her, and give you a son from her! Yea, I will bless her, and she shall*

*become a mother of nations; kings of people shall be from her*

*- Genesis 17:16p*

---

*God introduced himself as the spirit of conception in the beginning*

---

According to the Scriptures, the earth was characterized as a she. For example, in Genesis 4:11, the Lord said to Cain "the earth has opened her mouth to receive...." and it was also said in Psalm 67:6 that "he earth shall yield *her* increase". Base on the later example, one can infer that the earth possesses the attribute of a 'womb man' who could yield seeds. Have you ever stopped then to think that in the beginning, the earth was in a state of barrenness?

The womb of the earth out of which all good things, including man, came by was initially barren. The advent of the trees, the seas, vegetation, the animals, and even man proceeded out of a once-barren state. It is amazing to depict in Genesis, the book of the beginning, how God decided to begin "unafraid" when He began the beginning. God began with a challenge even in the beginning. Despite being God, He did not start out with satisfaction but was faced with a serious challenge. The raw material from which God would create all that is was void, empty, formless, and barren.

Who would have thought that something good could come out of such a barren state? God, however, was not perturbed by this situation (Genesis 1:2). The barrenness of mother earth did not panic Him—even though the earth was without form and void and the depths were covered with thick darkness. We can also liken this situation to a woman without a womb. I think that was just the state of the earth. It was a very critical case, a starting point of emptiness. Yet the barrenness of the earth was no hopeless case for God. After all, He had created mother earth, and her barrenness was for the birthing of newness. And what happened? Out of this barren earth that showed no sign of becoming fruitful, God brought forth life by the working of the Spirit of conception. God knew then and knows now exactly how to transform a barren womb into a producer of newness. God introduced Himself as the Spirit of conception in the beginning. What an introduction!

In other books of the Bible we find God introducing Himself as the *I am that I am,* as the lord of Hosts, as Yahweh, as El-shaddai, as Most High and many other names, but at the very beginning God introduces Himself as the fertility God, a creative life-giver who is able to

*Remember that this ability of God to bring new life out of barrenness is the first on His profile*

impregnate a barren womb, as One who can empower a wombless entity to birth remarkable newness. It is awesome to know this about God. Remember that this ability of God to bring new life out of barrenness is the first on His profile.

God chose to do this from the beginning so that we humans could understand that it is impossible for us, so far as God is concerned, not to reproduce. And so God began to show the way He has always produced life, even before the beginning began. Then He released the working of His Spirit to empower the earth and she conceives and brings forth. The Spirit of God had to move and brood upon mother earth before she could produce life. The working of His empowerment to conceive impregnated the earth and she bore all that made it become habitable for all living and non-living things today. He pronounced His Word, which is Spirit and Life, upon the earth. This Word ran very swiftly at His command in the beginning, as David described it in Psalm 147:15 and Psalm 148:5, to enable the earth to become a mother.

This act of His spirit first brooding over mother earth before her conception could take place was to tell that the God of heaven is also a God of preparation. He first and foremost prepared the womb of the earth for the blessings that was about to proceed from her. And so He paid the earth a visit by adequately preparing her womb for conception. This was what David meant in his memoir according to Psalm 65:9-10 that it was the Lord who visited the earth before it could conceive, as He also visited Sarah to become pregnant. He had to change the structure of her womb and made everything necessary ready in her womb to conceive.

The Lord prepared the earth for conception by watering its ridges abundantly, settling its furrows, softening its reproductive organs with showers, and above all blessed its growth that it might not suffer any miscarriage. God adequately prepared the earth for both her conception and safe deliveries.

Verse 9-10: "You visit the earth and water it, You greatly enrich it; The river of God is full of water; You provide their grain, for so You have prepared it. You water its ridges abundantly, You settle its furrows; You make it soft with showers, You bless its growth".

If God did not leave the earth in her barren state then rest assured that He will not leave you in a barren state, either. He will not be glorified if He leaves you in that condition and His purpose will not be accomplished. And if God did prepare the earth for conception and also did bless its growth for a safe delivery, then, God by His blessing upon you shall adequately prepare your ovaries, fallopian tube and uterus for your conception and a safe delivery. He will bless the growth of your baby's fertilization in your womb until you put to bed. He softened all the organs necessary for mother earth to experience a smooth gestation and delivery by His showers of blessing; and so shall He soften your organs by showering you with blessing to have a smooth conception and childbirth. As earlier said, God is a God of preparation and this fact is evident in many illustrations given in the Scriptures. One of them is the account in Isaiah 5:1-2 of His Beloved vineyard.

Verse 1: " .... My Well-beloved has a vineyard on a very fruitful hill."

Verse 2: "He dug it up and cleared out its stones, and planted it with the choicest vine. He built a tower in its midst, and also made a winepress in it; so He expected it to bring forth good grapes ...."

In this illustration, God has a vinyard on a fruitful hill which He is expecting good grapes from. Thus, He prepared it to achieve this purpose by digging it out (ploughed it), cleared out its stones, built in protective watchtower and made a winepress in it just for it to bring forth good grapes. He did not stop there as verse 6 of that chapter makes us know of His intention to always give rain (the blessing) for fruitfulness to take place. God did all these to see His expected fruits and I believe in the same manner, He carries out this operation on the woman to see His seeds come out of her. He alone can thoroughly prepare the womb by clearing out all the stones, briers, weeds and whatever it might be that wants to stop the woman from conceiving. For this reason, I will advise young ladies to make it part of their prayers; that God will thoroughly prepare their womb for conception and safe delivery, even as you are preparing for marriage. Don't wait until you are married before you start praying about it, do this and God will bless your womb for fertilization in marriage in the name of Jesus Christ. And for the married who are still expecting; and you have been told that there are stones or tumors present in your womb hindering conception, I pray that the God of preparation shall visit you. He would dig out all tumors and clear out the stones just for you to conceive in the name of Jesus Christ. Even if it requires Him to deploy His Spirit of burning and of judgment (Isaiah 4:4) to clear out all filth preventing your conception, He would do so to see His seeds come to earth. He will engage His Spirit to make the womb of the daughters of Zion holy for conception and their lives beautiful to His glory. He shall sweep out all the refuge of lies and judge the haughtiness of hindrances to your conception in Jesus name.

Remember, He also built in it a watchtower to protect the growth of the fruits of His Beloved vineyard, in the same way, I pray for you who always suffer miscarriage, that God shall have built in your womb protective watchtower for the baby(ies) in your womb until your safe delivery in the name of Jesus Christ. So He will do again what He did to the earth and His Vineyard and conceive in your life because He has a stake in creating you and in your Seeds. God has a stake in seeing the earth produce herbs, fruits, trees, grass, and seas because He has a plan in mind that must become factuality. This truth was established in Isaiah 45:18 that: "For thus says the Lord, who created the heavens, who is God, who formed the earth and made it, who has established it, *who did not create it in vain, who formed it to be inhabited*." He did not create the earth in vain when it was created at the beginning going by Genesis 1: 1 a. God had a plan for the earth to be inhabited and that is why He did not leave the earth in her acute state of barrenness. The earth rather receives blessing from God to bear useful herbs for its inhabitant (Hebrews 6:7).

Verse 7: "For the earth which drinks in the rain that often comes upon it and bears herbs useful for those by whom it is cultivated, receives blessing from God"

Just as the earth receives the blessing to produce fruits, you also need to receive the blessing to be able to produce mankind out of your flesh. It takes God's blessing and not so much of one's skillfulness in sexual activities. You also need the Spirit to move over the dark of your womb to conceive your kind, just as He moved over the face of the deep before mother earth could reproduce bounties.

Apart from the fact that God did not leave the earth in her barren state, He continued to bless the ground and its produce so that it cannot stop yielding. You will realize in Genesis 1 that after God creates a thing, it was recorded that *and God saw that it was good.* He sees them as *good* when He created them but saw them as *very good* after He pronounced the blessing upon all that He had created going by Genesis 1:31. His creation advanced from being marked good to very good after the blessing that will ensure they perform their purpose for creation. Not until His Spirit of blessing is poured upon them from on high, nothing becomes fruitful (Isaiah 32: 15).

Verse 15: "Until the Spirit is poured upon us from on high, and the wilderness becomes a fruitful field, and the fruitful field is counted as a forest".

This act of God is apparent in other many cases in the Bible. For example, the listing of blessing in Deuteronomy 28 accentuates His priority to bless everything living on earth both plant and creatures. He wants increase to take place perpetually from the ground, animals and humans, and so He established that the blessing on them will bring it about. It is the blessing that makes the fruit of the body happens. The same way the earth and plant require His showers of blessing to yield fruits (Ezekiel 34:26-27), so also do human require His showers of blessing to produce fruit of the body on earth. Here, God declared that He would cause His showers of blessings to rest; so that its recipient could yield her increase.

The earth who was once barren, had her birth-gate (womb)

eventually opened up after the move of the spirit of conception. The first fruits of the ground opened her womb and she yielded fruits each after its kind. Women are to also reproduce after its kind and have their birth-gate opened up by at least a firstborn. Everything God created had the blessing released on it to have at least their first fruits or firstborn on earth. The blessing sees to it that everything with a womb is opened first by a fruit/firstborn, according to God's design. This fact is clearly evident in the story of Pharaoh and the Egyptians, who at a particular time in history, had all their firstborn smitten—Exodus 12: 29-30.

"And it came to pass, that at midnight the Lord smote all the *firstborn* in the land of Egypt, from the *firstborn* of Pharaoh that sat on his throne unto the *firstborn* of the captive that was in the dungeon; and all the *firstborn* of cattle. And Pharaoh rose up in the night, he, and all his servants, and all the Egyptians; and there was great cry in Egypt; for there was not a house where there was not one dead".

This scripture, makes it clear to us that every creature in existence in the house of Pharaoh, including all his servants that lived down in dungeons, had a firstborn on earth. Despite that the Egyptians were not God's people, each of them, including all their captives, had their wombs opened by a firstborn. Should a people who reside in such unpleasant place as in the dungeon have the capacity to conceive children? If this breed of people who lived in such sorry state; and the Egyptians who were without God in their lives could have a firstborn; then you and I should be the most fortunate to conceive children, more so, in Christ Jesus. In Him, we have been blessed to become fruitful; hence our wombs must be opened at least by a first born among many. I discovered also from this story of Pharaoh and his Egyptian counterpart that for the first time, since the heart of Pharaoh had been hardened, that he saw a need for the pronouncement of blessing to regain all that was lost in the fight. According to the account of Exodus 12:32, after the decease of all the firstborns of the land; he eventually agreed that the Israelite should go and serve the Lord, and requested that Moses and Aaron should bless him also before embarking on the journey. This implies that Pharaoh to an extent, understood vividly, what the blessing could do in conception and the role it plays in bringing to earth the fruit of the body. He knew that the blessing on him could bring a restoration and reproduction of all the firstborns that had been lost.

So it is the blessings that open doors, open ways and open wombs. The doors or gates of any womb of His creation cannot be continually shut because by His design, it must open up and lift up its head to give way for new arrivals. The earth did not

*You are a sign of the introduction of a new beginning yet to unfold*

have hers continually shut because of the working of the Spirit upon her; and in the same way, your own womb gate shall not be shut continually, by the power of His Spirit working in you. The same manner the earth has been blessed or empowered to produce, the same way you shall become empowered to reproduce after your kind on earth.

We have seen how the barrenness of the earth ultimately led to the introduction of newness and new beginnings. This implies that your own condition, far from hopeless, is ripe for the introduction of new life on the earth. Some of us might resign ourselves to the fact that barrenness is a permanent state or even retire the possibility of conception. You cannot afford to resign or retire because unless you are as old as Sarah or the earth: you are too young to do so. You will be resigning or retiring too early, and this might be the reason you are not yet speaking with your children. The reality of your life will always be that you will become pregnant and carry your children. Do not forget that the promises of God are *Yea and Amen* concerning your becoming a mother and a father, and so do not retire rather revert to the Spirit of conception.

If out of barren earth came the blessings of light, seas, fruits and herbs for food, animals, and all living creature including man, then the creation is waiting for that blessing from your womb that will add color to our world. Just as a great bounty of blessings came out of mother earth after the Spirit of God worked upon her barrenness, so numerous blessing are about to come out of your womb because the working of the blessing of Sarah will be on you henceforth to see you become impregnated. I am certain that hope will shine in your seemingly hopeless case. Fulfillment is coming out of you, joy unspeakable and full of glory is coming out of you, and your blessed children will rise up to be a blessing to our world as were the Seeds of mother earth and the Seeds of Sarah. *Congratulations!*

You are a sign of the introduction of a new beginning yet to unfold. You are the proof that God has yet many new plans to execute before His coming, and your Seed is part of the instrument that will fulfill His plans for our world. What you are about to give birth to is precious, and that is why you are being shaken here and there, but do not be afraid, for God has visited you this time, and the working of His Spirit will work on you till you conceive. If He did not allow the earth to remain in her barren state, then, despite your condition, He will not let you remain there. Remember that in the beginning, the earth's barreness was a deadened case. Yet she became reproductive and remains so even all these thousands of years later—in her old age. Fruitfulness in old age is normal to God, because His principle of sowing and reaping transcends ages. As old as the earth is, she is still bearing fruits and several immeasurable things of great value to human existence are still from her womb till date; that is why we also cannot but bear fruit even at old age, as declared in Psalm 92:14.

Likewise, you, too, are about to give birth no matter what diagnosis you have been given. The fruit of your body will emerge regardless. The formation of the baby shall take place notwithstanding. The deadness of Sarah's womb made "natural" conception and childbearing impossible, but remember that the blessing of Sarah is spiritual and was from Heaven. So the deadness of her womb could not prevent her from receiving the blessing of conception, and your natural state cannot prevent your blessing, either.

With the engagement of the working Spirit of God, nothing about your case is impossible, no matter how dire it might seem. Therefore, fan your hope to a flame, even in the face of barrenness, because you shall become a mother in your lifetime. Barrenness can never be the final word! God's Word is the final word. If the blessing operates by the working of the Spirit of God as the Word of God teaches, then you cannot be stopped any more than mother earth could be stopped from bringing forth life by the will of God. Barrenness, like everything else in the universe, submits to the highest power. Barrenness in the body or in the land is a fertile field for the inception of a new beginning with God. It is a fading point for the state of barrenness and a feeding point for new eras for fruitfulness and multiplication. So, welcome to another era of the baby boom!

God has used many cases, including that of the earth, to reveal to us emphatically that the state of barrenness for Him is an opportunity for launching a new status and bringing forth life. It is another avenue again of creating out of nothing. Though this may be contrary to how human beings see it, we are wise if we come to see things as God sees them. When God sees a barren body or a barren land, He sees as new opportunity for His life–spawning act. Henceforth, see that body or that land as a medium for showcasing God's own newness, and it shall soon become the reality of your life.

Make this your daily confession, and you will always attract the working of the Spirit of the blessing of the womb that will launch your life and your family into newness.

# Scriptural Notes

➢ Genesis 1: la, 2, 31

➢ Genesis 4: 11

➢ Exodus 12: 29-30, 32

➢ Deuteronomy 28: 1-14

➢ Psalm 65: 9-10

➢ Psalm 67: 6

➢ Psalm 92: 14

➢ Psalm 147: 15; 148: 5

➢ Isaiah 4: 4

➢ Isaiah 5: 1-2, 6

➢ Isaiah 32: 15

➢ Ezekiel 34: 26-27

➢ Hebrews 6: 7

# CHAPTER FIVE

*The Bitter Water Causing Fibroid Tumors, Barrenness,*
*and Miscarriages in Women*

*And I will bless her, and give you a son from her! Yea, I will bless her, and she shall*

*become a mother of nations, kings of people shall be from her*

*- Genesis 17:16p*

---

*Know that for every*
*unnecessarily lingering*
*battle, there is a cause*

---

The blessing of Sarah supersedes all obstructions to giving birth, including all curses. It is a mystery that the church is yet to unfold. Dr. David Oyedepo has declared in one of his teachings that the blessings of God are the cure for every curse. I completely agree. Let us examine why by looking at what happened in the beginning when God created the first man and woman.

When Adam and Eve were first created in the image of God, He first of all pronounced the blessing upon them to enable them to become fruitful, and that is why the blessing He had already pronounced upon them while they were spirit (Genesis 1:27-28) began working on them when He eventually formed them into bodily beings from the dust in Genesis 2:7. Both of them were naturally productive because the blessing was upon both the man and the "man with the womb" Eve.

God told them (just as he later told Abraham and Sarah), "I will bless you, and you will become fruitful and multiply. Yea, I will bless you and you will subdue the earth and have dominion over every living thing on the earth." Now we know that God is a great God, and He is a consistent God, who does not in any way contradict Himself. His sequence of first pronouncing the blessing on every living thing He created was evidenced even after He created the fishes, the birds, and all living creatures (Genesis 1: 21-22). Despite the fact these creatures are not human beings, the blessing had to be pronounced in order for all of them to become fruitful and multiply and fill the seas and the earth down to this very day.

This same blessing that God pronounced upon these non-human living things has made it impossible for female animals, birds, and fishes not to procreate down to this day. It has been impossible to see any female mammal, reptiles, birds, etc., who was incapable of becoming pregnant. Since this blessing was pronounced upon these creatures, it became impossible also for the male not to be productive and feed. Males will always impregnate their females (Deuteronomy 7:14), and they will always have food to eat because the blessing is working on them, too.

Verse 14: "Thou shalt be blessed above all people: there shall be no male or female barren among you, or *among your cattle*".

They, like father Abraham, do not lack and they, like mother Sarah, will always give birth no matter what because the blessing is working. That is why we can afford to buy food for our domestic animals at home whether horses, dogs, cats, pigs, hens, or birds. Sometimes when we wake up in the morning, before even feeding ourselves, we first go and give them their food and water and at night feed them again before we can go to bed. Why is this so? It is because the blessing is working on their lives and so they cannot lack food to eat.

Even if you do not give them food, once they go out to play on the street, food will be placed somewhere by someone for them, simply because the blessing is working on them. This was what Jesus implied when He taught His disciples that they should not worry at all about what to eat or what to drink or about what clothes to put on because the blessing from the Father would always ensure they have those things (Matthew 6:25-26). So He went further to expound on the workings of that blessing by bidding them to look at the birds of the air, who neither sow nor reap yet the blessing of the Father ensure that they are fed, and consider how much more blessed indeed they are as beings created in the image of the Father. Another interesting example is that of Leviticus 25:20-21. Here, God said to Moses that perhaps he and the Israelite with him are worried about "what shall we eat in the seventh year, since we shall not sow nor gather in our produce?" that He will command His blessing on them, to bring forth produce enough for three years. It was by His blessing on them that they could bring forth more than enough produce in the sixth year.

When the blessing is working, man or woman cannot lack any good thing. *The blessing is an empowerment to possess, an empowerment to prosper, an empowerment to conceive, an empowerment to impregnate, an empowerment to fertilize, an empowerment to manifest* whatever your heart desires so long as it is in accordance with His Will and timing for your life. So from the beginning everything God created was productive–both the first man and woman and the first male and female creature of every species. They were empowered to become whatever God wanted them to become.

## TWO SEPARATE CURSES ON THOSE PRONOUNCED AS ONE!

The blessing was working on the first man and the first woman until the fall when the curses were pronounced. God never had the reason to curse anything He created until Adam and Eve sinned against Him, resulting in His pronouncing a curse on each of them. That is, He pronounced a separate curse on the man and on the woman–meaning there were two curses on the man and woman He had declared to be one . Note that in the beginning it was not so. He pronounced the blessing upon both of them and not a different blessing on each of them. Only after the fall of the first man and woman did God have a curse to pronounce separately upon man and woman whom He loved and had a plan of fulfillment for. Compare this with the case of Abram and Sarai. Despite all the blessing He had already pronounced upon Abram and working on him, He had (because of the curse) to pronounce the blessing separately on Sarai in order to enable her to conceive. If He had not, she could not have become fruitful.

Someone may wonder why the other women besides Sarah were able to conceive easily in those days and day despite the fact that the blessing was not pronounced on them. You may also think that the curse that was pronounced upon the first woman, Eve, was not the curse of barrenness, so why did the blessing have to be pronounced upon Sarah before she could conceive? These are good questions! And I will try to do justice to both in this chapter. Please patiently walk along with me in this chapter to see where barrenness, miscarriages, and fibroid tumors emanated from.

When God cursed Adam (Genesis 3:17), the curse can be summed up in one word: Poverty. Meanwhile he had pronounced a separate curse on the woman, which can be summed up as: Related to childbirth. The curse on the woman has to do with sorrowful conception and painful delivery (Genesis 3:16). This curse, however, includes enmity between the serpent and the woman and also enmity between her Seed and the serpent's seed. Although the curse of hostility between the serpent and the woman and between the serpent's seed and the woman's Seed was pronounced on the serpent and not on the woman, it has a great effect on the woman. If you study your Bible carefully, you will realize that the woman's Seed is written with a capital letter *S* while the serpent's seed is written with a small letter *s*, and this is how the woman's problems got compounded (Genesis 3:15).

Verse 15: "And I will put enmity between you and the woman, and between your seed and her Seed; He shall bruise your head, and you shall bruise His heel".

Verse 16: "To the woman He said; I will greatly multiply your sorrow and your conception; in pain you shall bring forth children; your desire shall be for your husband, and he shall rule over you".

Verse 17: "Then to Adam He said; because you have heeded

the voice of your wife, and have eaten from the tree of which I commanded you, saying, 'you shall not eat of it': cursed is the ground for your sake; in toil you shall eat of it all the days of your life".

The serpent, of course, was the devil, and his seed are the demons. The Seed of the woman, however, are the children of light who would be born to bruise the head of the devil himself and his demons. These are the Seeds of promise, not ordinary seeds, and Jesus is part of this Seed. Seeing that the curse on him was always to be at hostility with the woman and her Seed and thus a threat to his works, the devil decided to try to gain the upper hand by making sure the woman's Seed were not even born in the first place. It is most likely that Satan got a hint to God's redemptive plan for man at the mention of the curse about the woman's Seed bruising his head. And since then, there was a declaration of war against the woman and her seeds.

Besides, the devil has been against God's idea of creating man from day one, more so making man a co-creator with Him. So he capitalized on the curse related to childbirth! We have no idea of the depth of change and chaos caused by the declaration of these curses. Satan seriously took the advantage of the pronouncement of the curse and enlarged it progressively. Thus, when he sees a Seed that will come to the earth to bruise his head, he fights hard and does his best to make sure the woman does not give birth to that Seed in the first instance. How do I know? Check it in Bible history. You will find that most of the women who were barren were those who were to carry great Seed that comes to manifest God's plan on the earth and sends the devil trembling. These are the children whom God has separated to subdue the earth and be used for His own glory.

Consider Sarah: She was to bring forth the Seed of promise (a model nation) according to God's plan, and this makes the devil trembling. Isaac's wife Rebekah was barren because the promise of nations coming out of Abraham was about to be fulfilled in her son Jacob (Genesis 25:21-23), and this was a threat to the devil because he hates nations as much as he hates families and individuals. Jacob's wife Rachel was barren because she was to bring forth a Seed named Joseph whose existence was to break the record of kings coming out of Abraham (Genesis 30). Samson's mother was barren because she was to carry a Seed that would be mighty on the earth to judge the seeds of the devil (Judges 13). Hannah, too, was barren because she was to give birth to Samuel, a Seed that God would use to make the ears of others tingle and instruct His people. John the Baptist's mother, Elizabeth, was barren for she was to carry a seed that would prepare the way for the One who would destroy the works of the devil and his seeds, and so the war to prevent His birth was intense.

Mary the mother of Jesus could not be stopped because she was already blessed so that she might give birth to the Saviour. How do I know? The angel Gabriel, who stood in the presence of God daily watching Him pronounce blessing, told Mary, "Blessed are you among women." Angel Gabriel saw it when God was blessing Mary in heaven to dispel all obstruction on the way of the coming King and so when he came to deliver God's message to her, he could not but mention the fact that according to their heavenly pattern and activities, she had just been pronounced blessed among women (Luke 1:19-28). And therefore her Seed could not be stopped because the mother (Mary) was already blessed in heaven without her asking for this blessing of the womb.

## THE SEVERITY OF THE CURSES

The hostility against Woman became severe and intense since the curse. That is why to this day many women still die in the course of childbirth, some suffer miscarriages which are same as sorrowful conceptions, some are barren, some are afflicted with fibroid tumors, and with cancers of the breast and of the womb and other diseases. These are the products of the enmity against the woman. God does not have a reason to pronounce curses if not for the devil that incite His people against Him so he could always have a basis for fighting them. Infliction of curses such as *"No birth, No pregnancy, No conception, having miscarrying womb and dry breasts"* were punishments for enmity with God as seen in Hosea 9:11&14 *(NKJV)*. All of these moves are part of his plan to prevent the Seed of the woman from being born.

Have you ever seen a man with a fibroid tumor of the stomach? I have not, though I have seen men deep in poverty and want. The curse is at work, but the devil exploits the curse related to childbirth to fight hard against women and their seed. The entire climate of occurrences around the woman changed since Satan began capitalizing on the curse. But thank God for Christ who came and handcuff all curses to the cross so that the women could conceive His Seeds and men could become rich. Even though the woman was deceived, the verdict remains that she shall be saved in child bearing in Christ Jesus (1Timothy 2:14-15). More so, the woman's seed has been empowered to bruise his head.

For the same reason, the devil is still fighting women because he is afraid of their Seeds. The reason he seems to succeed at this sometimes is that the curse was already pronounced; and the curse is the basis he stands upon and uses as an opportunity to sow havoc. This was also what he wanted to do to Job when God gave him permission to touch him. He tried to seize and maximize the opportunity to kill Job because he was threatened and uncomfortable with Job's existence. Remember Satan's response to God's boastings of Job? That "have you not built a hedge around him, around his household, and around all that he has on every side?" going by Job 1:10. This statement simply shows that he had been trying in the past to attack Job but God's hedges around him and his belongings made Job impenetrable. God already knew that the devil could expand the mere permission He had been given to touch Job's *belongings* to touch his *life* (that is, kill him), and that is why God kept stressing to him not to touch his life (see Job 1:12 and Job 2:6).

Despite the fact that he had used the permission God gave him to kill all 10 of Job's children and destroy all his belongings, the devil was still not satisfied. He went back to God and said, "Let me touch Job himself," and God again told him not to touch Job's life (Job 2). Why? Because God already saw the end from the beginning and knew that all the devil had been actually looking for is an opportunity to kill Job himself and so He kept telling him "do not tamper with his life." This is the same thing the devil is doing with women through the ages—fighting more than necessary and aggravating the curse of mere pain during childbirth until we find women dying in childbirth, having repeated miscarriages, and afflicted with wicked diseases that prevent conception and childbirth. So he engineers all these because in the beginning it was not so.

# FIBROID TUMORS

Let us examine another curse causing fibroid tumors and barrenness from the scriptural account of Numbers 5:11-28 which the devil also capitalizes on to increasingly afflict women today. See what some of the verses reads;

Verse 11-13: "And the Lord spoke to Moses, saying", Speak to the children of Israel, and say to them: if any man's wife goes astray and behaves unfaithfully towards him, and a man lies with her carnally, and it is hidden from the eyes of her husband, and it is concealed that she has defiled herself, and there was no witness against her or was she caught"

Verse 16-22: "And the priest shall bring her near and set her before the Lord. The priest shall take holy water in an earthen vessel, and take some of the dust that is on the floor of the tabernacle and put it into the water...... And the priest shall put her under oath, and say to the woman, "if no man has lain with you, and if you have not gone astray to uncleanness while under your husband's authority, be free from this bitter water that brings a curse. But if you have gone astray while under your husband's authority, and if you have defiled yourself and some man other than your husband has lain with you"..... the Lord make you a curse and an oath among your people, when the Lord makes your thigh rot and your *belly swell;* and may this water that causes the *curse go into your stomach, and make your belly swell* and your thigh rot."

Verse 27-28: "When he has made her drink the water, then it shall be, if she has defiled herself and behaved unfaithfully toward her husband, that the water that brings a curse will enter her and become bitter, and her belly will swell, .... but if the woman has not defiled herself, and is clean, then *she shall be free* and *may conceive children"*

From the illustration given in the verses, it shows that fibroid tumors have been in existence ages ago and that it is nothing new under the sun. It was formerly known as the bitter water that causes swollen belly in women but is now what medical scientist named fibroid. Once upon a time, in the life of the Israelite, any woman found going aside from her husband to lay with other men becomes guilty and liable to drink of the bitter water that causes the curse. When this bitter water that causes the curse enters into her bowels, it will make her belly swell (verse 22) profusely. The woman henceforth becomes a curse among her people and would not be able to conceive seed (verse 27-28). The swollen belly prevents the seed of her husband from staying and germinating in her womb. By the conclusion drawn from this analogy in verse 28, the presence of the bitter water in her belly hinders conception. It therefore implies that the bitter water is a disease in the womb that prevents conception from taking place.

Meanwhile, exactly this is what fibroid does in women today. Fibroid equally makes the woman's belly to swell and this prevent conception of seeds. Medical scientist only gave it a new name other than the bitter water causing the curse of swollen turgidity in women's belly. Since it is called bitter water, one could tell that its make up is of a watery substance, as it is for fibroid. Actually, fibroid is a watery substance that can dissolve but becomes a solid substance over time in women if left untreated. It will first take the form of water before solidifying into tumors that result in swelling belly. This is an outcome of uncontrollably fleshly pleasures according to the Numbers 5, contrary to general belief that it is resulting from long abstinence from sexual act.

Basically, from the scriptural view, fibroid is explained as the consequence of a woman passing through so many hands sexually. This scripturally established truth cannot be contested that worldly pleasures could attract and reactivate curses once written against women, working contrary to them, and standing in their way to conceiving. However, we know that there are some exceptional cases which are not resulting from sexual actions but from spiritual battles. How do I mean?

Somewhere in Mathew 13:24-30, Jesus gave an insightful parable about the sudden appearance and growth of a weed in the place of good seed. From this parable, He said while men slept, his enemy came and sowed weeds among seeds. This account tells us that whenever we find unwanted things growing in a supposedly good and fertile ground, it becomes an enemy has done this event.

The enemy here is Satan, the devil. In today's contemporary world, we perceive a lot of things happening to women as normal. For example, some see miscarriages as being a normal part of woman's life, and same as fibroid. Meanwhile, Jesus has not changed His stand on the fact that these are part of the done deeds of the enemy, for in the beginning, they were not so. As the world becomes contemporary and sophisticated, we cannot overlook the fact that the devil has gone contemporary and sophisticated too in running his system of evil perpetrations. He continues to enforce the curses with a special focus on deceiving the woman to sin. You know he always look for a basis to lay down a blanket of curses for the woman and the only way for the curse to stand is through a justified cause–Sin and ignorance. Though the death of Jesus came to wipe out all curses and ordinances working contrary to our lives; sin was not wiped out from the earth. Truly He bore our sins on the cross but sin itself, which is the cause of a curse, remains in existence. Sins, however, shall not have dominion over us but can still attract, enforce or reactivate curses if careless; and the devil employ this strategy a lot in today's world, capitalizing on people's ignorance.

---

*You should not be indulging in sexual intercourse or dining activities while sleeping*

## DINNING AND SEXUAL ACTIVITIES WHILE MEN SLEPT

Besides, the system he is running now is also such that transcends him just capitalising on the causes of the curse. Since the woman had always been his target for deception and destruction; he has introduced several other operational strata that trigger entry of curses through openings such as even when men and women slept and slept off in spirit.

It is amazing to know that some women in this age notice that while they slept, they eat in their dreams. Some others noticed that they do have sexual dealings in dreams too. These are prevailing occurrences contrary to the scriptures. They were occurrences I believe were not happening to men and women who lived ages ago, aside from Peter, whom the Lord wanted to correct about his discrimination against the Gentiles being a Jew. Otherwise, any of such event outside His influence, would be much the same as having fellowship with demons. These are part of what Jesus referred to as an enemy has done this while men slept. They are part of Satan's operational devices introduced to prevent His seeds from coming to earth. Females engaging in such dinning and sexual activities while they slept literally create an opening for the implantations of unwanted seeds (weeds of tumors) in the belly which could also result in miscarriages.

Going by the study of the Word, I realized in over seventy verses where dream was mentioned, that dreams were used mostly by God to issue warning (Abimelech, Laban, Pharaoh ...) or give direction Joseph, the spouse of Mary) or mostly to reveal/pre- inform about the occurrence of a future event Joseph in Egypt, Jacob, Nebuchadnezzar, Pontius Pilate's wife ... ). Dreams and visions were intended by God to serve as part of His medium of communicating with man. The only person in the Bible who had a different opinion about dreams was Solomon who concluded that they are usually resulting from the multitude of the day's business. It is however not surprising to have such view from a man who had numerous dinning and sexual activities with a confederation of women in his lifetime. I know from experience that God speaks to His own people at times through visions and dreams, to help them know what to do, and which way is best to walk, but I doubt if He has such time as to be orchestrating a replay of individual's daily activities to them in dreams. Dreams and visions are a powerful tool and I have been privileged to enjoy tremendous access to information before they ever happen on earth, as a result, which has contributed in giving me an unprecedented movement in life along the right direction. In the same manner, some are manifesting a terrible and frustrating life because of the unpleasant experiences they have while they slept. This is contrary to God's design for the purpose intended for dreams and visions and the architect of these unpleasant experiences is the wicked one.

These displeasing activities in dream, have created openings for the implantation of fibroid in some women's womb today. Majority of these women cannot explain how they came about fibroid tumors in their wombs. We must not be ignorant of the enemy's latest devices and so women must fight to stop these events. Stopping these experiences from re-occurring requires giving one's life to Jesus Christ and being dedicated to Him. If you have done so and still have such persisting in your life; then you need to engage the weapon of fasting and prayer for its banishment.

You should not be indulging in sexual intercourse or dining activities while sleeping. Jesus said this kind do not go away except by fasting and prayer. When it does not look His kind that is happening, then it is automatically this kind. This kind of occurrences is contrary to His kind, and therefore requires uprooting by fasting and prayer. As you fast and pray, this kind of experiences in your life will stop and every other source of bitter water causing the curse in your life shall be cut off. The living water from His throne will enter into your body system; flush Out all wicked plantations and also do a thorough work of purging, cleansing and rejuvenation on all affected areas in the name of Jesus Christ.

## PROLONGED BATTLES THROUGH COVENANT

The other of his introductions that he capitalises on to prevent the woman's seed from coming to earth is the reactivation of covenants made by forefathers. It is possible that there was a time one's ancestors did enter into some strange and inimical covenants that continuously seek compliance from off springs from one generation to another. Some ancestors even invoke curses upon their family lineage through initiations and perpetrations of evil acts during their lifetime. These initiations have obligations that are sometimes to be fulfilled by offsprings who on default would be compelled to face the music. These are part of the sin of the fathers that are being paid for by the children. These misdeeds and iniquities are presently affecting the children; and putting a barrier on their way to enjoying their lives through barrenness. Some of these fathers did actually covenant with altars that are actively sustaining all oath made upon it till date. This is not to scare you but know that for every unnecessarily lingering battle, there is a cause. The cause could be covenants or altars seeking compliance with or fulfillment of obligations. These unseen battles are the causes of some couples' delay today, as I have been privileged to hear of such cases. However, God is the Most High, who will help you by His mercies and deliver your miracles into your hands.

There is no smoke without a fire up. For every prolonged battle you are facing in life, there is always an altar powering, fueling and sustaining that battle. An altar is usually the main power house and not agents assigned from these altars. Every armory used by the agents assigned from an altar is gotten from the altar, hence, rather than focusing on the agents assigned to hinder you, focus on destroying the altar instead. Destroy the altar sustaining the battle; because once that altar is rendered powerless, the battle is ended. The altar is strengthening the battles and so the altar needs pulling down. This was what Jesus knew and understood that made Him not to cease crying aloud and again (Mathew 27:46 & 50-51) to the

Father until when. He saw the veil of the temple (altar) was rented into two from top to bottom, with nothing standing. The temple was rendered useless and powerless since then and that is why He knew that it was finished. All barriers, obstructions, hindrances, inaccessibility were finished and ended.

The goodnews is that for every work of the enemy, Jesus' appearance has brought a commensurate counter measures. A counter measure that frees the children from the sins of their fathers by His blood and His mercies. A counter measure that exempts the children from fulfilling obligations on the behalf of their fathers by His death on the cross, He already paid them off so that you do not have to pay again. So if you are Christ's, rather than panicking and praying without focus, search yourself and search out your family history, then, in that light approach God with a loud cry to rent down all altars sustaining lingering battles in your life in the name of Jesus Christ. The renting of the temple took place while Jesus was on the cross to die for you and I; and if truly life replaced death, and blessing replaced curses at the cross, then the cross stands today as a witness against all altars reactivating curses in your life in the name of Jesus Christ. Begin to issue counter decrees and press into prophetic pronouncements and the blessing to break free from all entanglement. If you are yet to accept Christ, I will advise that you should give your life to Him today so that He can rescue you from all curses or else I cannot guarantee your freedom. Jesus is the only way out and your only way out of this present family reproach.

Run now to Him because He alone is our advocate with the Father and can plead for His mercies over you as His new offspring. His blood alone can avail for you, none else. Approaching God in this light and accordingly will draw the attention of heaven to you for the blessing of the womb. Remember He alone can bless our curses just like He alone has the power to turn curses into blessings (Deutronomy 23:5 & Nehemiah 13:2) as He did for the Israelite. There is an authority and power vested in the name of Jesus Christ, and that name can do and undo if you call on Him. And in the name of Jesus Christ your soul is saved from death and your life will be grafted in Him. As you have decided to surrender to Jesus, the benefits of calling upon that name will show forth in your life henceforth.

I pray for you with a confirmed case of fibroid, that the fibroid tumors will turn out a baby in your womb, and shall work together for your testimony in the name of Jesus Christ! The God who creates something out of nothing will form your baby in your womb out of the fibroid tumors, if you believe. Fibroid is an invader, it is like a chaff contending with the appearance of a wheat that is the real thing. I pray that every implantation of weed and chaff in your womb shall be rooted out in Jesus name. The chaff however is nothing before the wheat says the almighty as declared in Jeremiah 23:28. And so, I pray that all fibroid be rendered as nothing before the fertilisation of your baby in the name of Jesus Christ. Who says fibroid and a baby cannot co-exist? Isaiah 11:6 says, a time will come that "the wolf shall dwell with the lamb, and the leopard shall lie down with a young goat ... and a little child shall lead them". This implies that even though your baby and fibroid co-exist, your little baby will lead in this contest for occupancy.

Fibroid cannot stand His blessing of conception, and therefore from today, it shall give way for the legal owner and rightful occupant of your womb in the name of Jesus Christ. In Isaiah 27:4,

God said "who can set briers and thorns against Him in battle? For He will go through them and would burn them off together or else they should make peace with Him". God cannot be boxed! He will always go through the obstruction for His production to take place. Because He alone has the power to bring a clean thing out of an unclean (Job 14:4); out of that same womb where fibroid is said to be present shall emerge babies. He will bring sweetness out of this rock for you (Psalm 81:16). He shall set before you a table of blessing of the womb in the presence of your enemies. That fibroid will turn to a fine boy (girl), if you believe. Operating fibroid may cause an irreparable damage to the uterus which then lessens the chances for conception or cut short your life.

Hence do not let the presence of a fibroid in your womb bother you, it shall wither away and melt down so that your baby whom God already called blessed shall appear for manifestation, in the name of Jesus Christ. Because your seeds are already pronounced blessed, they have been empowered to shove fibroid aside for its own appearance, and so shall your experience be. The Spirit of Life Creation would bring you health and cure in the name of Jesus Christ. He will undo them all for His name sake, and because He has a stake in your children, He will change the structure and condition of your womb just to see you conceive. The battle is His and not yours; so He is able to rid them out for you without Him applying a pin on your flesh. Rather than focusing on that fibroid, look to Jesus who is the Life giver and has handcuffed all tumors to the cross thousands of years ago. Hence, ignore that fibroid because it is not the main issue for your conception to take place. God is able to raise up children to Abraham from these stones of tumors (Matthew 3:9). Believe it and you shall soon testify that your babies were conceived after all!

## MISCARRIAGE

Miscarriage is another issue that needs to be addressed from the scriptural point of view and this chapter would be incomplete without it. It seemed another operational devise that the enemy uses to prevent the seeds of the woman from coming to earth. Though miscarriage might be a contemporary trend now amongst women; God's stand about it has not changed. No matter how much people perceive of it as normal, it is not the truth of God's plan for women. His thought (plan) towards you are good (not evil) and of peace; to give you an expected end of a safe delivery (Jeremiah 29:11). He wants to reveal to you the abundance of truth (Jeremiah 33:6) on this matter and the truth you know and understand will set you free from suffering miscarriage. His promise is that you shall not conceive nor bring forth children for trouble (Isaiah 65:23). God did not knit together that baby in your womb to be lost through miscarriage as they do not waste their resources in heaven. The doctors have told you that it is caused by stress or undertaking tedious task but scriptural account begs to differ with this theory.

If there are any set of people who had experienced stress in its fullest measures, they were the women of Israel in those days. These women lived under affliction. They sleep under heavy bondage and wake up to hard labour for four hundred years, yet they never suffered miscarriage. Despite their inhuman living conditions and having to journey on foot through the wilderness too, they multiplied and continued giving birth to children in the process. They trekked endless miles without any access to aids or ambulance supports to help cushion the effect of stress, yet, the scriptures record it that they increased and multiplied in the land.

These women probably were sleeping on the ground or at best had their backs lain on woods, still there was no room for miscarriages in their lives. How? God's blessing!

The blessing of God was the babies' stay in their wombs. This was what David articulated in Psalm 22: 9-10 & Psalm 71: 6 about how that God participated in his conception and delivery. Here, he said; "By You I have been upheld from birth ... " "But You (God) are He who took me out of the womb .... I was cast upon You from birth, from my mother's womb You have been My God". That God had been his bedrock and stay from his mother's womb was evident in his life's experiences. I am sure there were stern attempts to prevent baby David from being conceived but for God who was with him from his mother's womb, he came to life. Even after he was conceived, there must have been directed complications to thrust him out of the womb but for His God again; he was safely delivered. David knew and understood that his successful conception and delivery had the hand of his God in it. If it had not been God who was his stay and took him out of the womb, he would probably not have come to earth.

Just as David's delivery involved the hand of God taking him out of the womb, so also was that of Isaac and John's. Sarah and Elizabeth must have been aided by the unbeatable One to have successfully put to bed in their condition. These two women were recorded to be very old of age and could hardly push a baby through but for God's intervention. His hand must have assisted them in having a smooth and safe childbirth in the absence of gynecologist. He who causes to conceive alone has the unlimited ability to successfully bring to the time of delivery (Isaiah 66:9); so why not cast your baby's delivery on Him even while it is still in the womb. Only God can oversee activities going on in the womb for a safe delivery, and not so much of one's carefulness during the period of pregnancy.

Besides, God's innumerable company of angels created to minister to the heirs of salvation will not watch you lose that baby to the enemy contesting with its arrival into the earth. From my study of the Word, I realised that God has uncountable number of angels actively working because He has a stake in the heirs to inherit salvation. He assigns an angel to each child about to come earth to see them through their journeys from the womb to the earth, and eventually to help lead them to the Lord Jesus Christ. Seeing that they are the ones to continue His reign over the earth, He does everything to bring them here safely. This truth is apparent in the story of Mary and Elizabeth, where we see all angel assigned to each of them just for the sake of the babies in their womb. This is also evident in the story of the woman spoken of in Revelation 12. She was about to give birth and there was a contest for the arrival of the child but the angels were deployed to save the situation.

In the same light, I believe it was the innumerable company of angels assigned to the children of Israel that were their saving grace from the heavy burdens they were subjected to in Egypt. The angels were actively on duty to put in force their conception and delivery despite Pharaoh's strategies against their seeds. The same angels must have aided Sarah to have had a smooth gestation and delivery. Angels exist because of us and our children about to come. They were created to minister to that seed in your womb, so involve them in your conception and delivery rather than thinking it is by might. When your angels are in charge, you cannot suffer miscarriage because their Master has a stake in what is about to come out of you.

See what God Himself said about miscarriage in Exodus 23:25. He said "so you shall serve the Lord your God and He will *bless* ..." Bless? Bless? Bless! Again!!! This is God Himself speaking here–about blessing them and their intakes to prevent sickness, miscarriage, and barrenness. He said it is the blessing that He would employ, to see that none of them suffers miscarriage. That is to say, His blessing on them will ensure that nothing whatsoever would be strong enough to thrust their seeds out of their womb. He said "there shall nothing cast their young" *KJV*.

God's blessing is wonderful, isn't it? I mean: it is full of wonders. He did not stop there; He also emphasized the fact that this blessing on them would exclude them all from barrenness in the land. He however, puts a condition.

His condition is serving the Lord your God and the question is, how many are still serving the Lord their God after marriage? Some couples easily settle for the comfort of marriage and seized to be actively involved in serving God as before marriage. The wife's excuse becomes "I am married so I cannot come" while the husband's reason for absenteeism in the service of His Lord is "I am now with a bride and I cannot come". It is a good thing and I am not against being with your spouses, but when being in the presence of our spouses begins to take precedence over being in His presence and in His service, that you cannot suffer miscarriage may not be a pledge.

Do not be wise in your own eyes because God cannot be

*His blessing on them would not allow them go out of the womb before their time*

mocked. His blessings are exclusively reserved for those who will serve Him with the whole of their heart, their soul, their might, their strength, with their lives and to whom He will show mercy. I want to share with you an example of a couple I have always admired. I knew this couple at the prayer meeting of the Watch force intercessory unit of Daystar Christian Centre, the Church where I belong in Nigeria. This couple lifestyle excites me and I admire them so much because of their consistency in serving the Lord through prayers and intercession. This couple are both medical doctors and I have been seeing them regularly attending weekly prayer meetings, monthly vigils, and even yearly retreats before they got married.

After they wedded, I noticed they did not stop coming to pray; and intercede for others in spite of their busy shifts as medical practitioners. Sometimes, I see the couple holding hands into the prayer venue and my heart leaps in awe for their commitment. Having seen them regularly for some time after marriage without a child, I knew they were experiencing a delayed conception, still they did not stopped coming to pray. Then one day, it dawned or me that I have never prayed for this couple in my closet regarding their conception. But the Holy Spirit reminded me of their commendable level of commitment and that without praying, for them, they are blessed and shall soon be speaking with their children. And truly it happened, as I was glad the day I saw the wife pregnant and they are just blessed today. This exemplary lifestyle I believe should be the attitudes of mothers and fathers to be towards the service of the Most High.

I always count it a big privilege serving Him; it has always been my pleasure to do so and I pray that nothing will stop me because therein lies my joy, strength, blessing, and fulfillment. I have tried other things and they never fetched me what His reward programme have granted me thus far, and that makes it too late for me to act otherwise. We are created to serve Him-for we are for His pleasure. Seek God, when you genuinely look for God, you will find babies in the process.

On a final note on what God has to say concerning miscarriage is in Isaiah 27:3&6. From this account, God gave a description of a fruitful vine that produces red wine which can be likened to a woman that produces babies. He said in verse 3 that:

*"I the Lord will keep it; I will water it every moment: lest any hurts it, I will keep it night and day".* God is painting a picture here of how He watches over a fruitful womb to ensure a maturity unto delivery. Invariably, He is saying to pregnant women that it shall come to pass that He will keep your pregnancy and water it every moment lest any should hurt it. He will regularly bless it, lest it be trusted out of its place. He said that He would also keep it at night and day so that the enemy's dart will not cast the young seed out of the womb. And He concluded in verse 6 that these seeds would bud, take root and blossom by His workings until the face of the world is filled with fruits. It is by these workings of His Spirit of conception that we can have a similar experience like that of Elizabeth whom the Bible records in Luke 1:57 that: when Elizabeth's *full time* came to be delivered, she brought forth a son. His own workings and involvement ensures that you experience a full time gestation

period: not a quarter time or half time gestation period that is prevalent in our world today. God is showing us how that He commits Himself to ensuring that the fruits of our body come to fill the world through His acts of regularly watching over them, blessing them in the womb, making them take root and blossom until their delivery into the earth.

Besides, your Heavenly Father who causes conception is capable of also bringing to the time of birth. Just as He has declared in Isaiah 66:9 that "shall He bring to the time of birth and not cause delivery and shall He who causes delivery shut up the womb?". No way! He is more than able to pull your baby through to the time of birth and cause your safe delivery too.

You can see how your children shall fill the world by the help of your Father in heaven and not by your own carefulness or avoiding stress. It is the Father's work to make the baby stay in the womb until its full time to be delivered. His blessing on them would not allow them go out of the womb before their due time of appearance on earth. I pray today, that the Lord God of hosts shall be the stay of your baby in your womb in the name of Jesus Christ. He shall strengthen the bars of your womb gates and bless your children within you (Psalm 147:13). No more shall miscarriage be named with you in the name of Jesus Christ. Make this Isaiah 27 your confession and prayer and I can assure you, you will see your children fill the world. Also make Luke 1:57 your daily confession during gestation period; and your full time of delivery shall come through, in the name of Jesus Christ. Your salvation is nearer to you now than ever if you will consider these things and do them.

## REVERSING THE CURSE

All these calamities wrought by the devil did God foresaw, that He decided to reverse the order, by always pronouncing His blessings on individual women, who could harness His blessings in Christ to nullify every curse on her pathway to becoming a mother. And so He started out with Sarah, the mother of all living, just as He started with Abraham, the father of blessing. He then replaced Adam with Abraham and Eve with Sarah, so that we could now call Abraham and not Adam our father; and Sarah not Eve our mother, because they were blessed like the first man and first woman when they had not sinned. So we have been asked to look to Abraham, our father and to Sarah our mother, who bore us through faith according to Isaiah 51:2. They are being called to the blessings and not to curses. Eve used to be referred to as the mother of all living according to Genesis 3:20, but due to the fall, she was replaced by Sarah, whom we now call the mother of all living and also being referred to as the mother of us all in the faith (Galatians 4:22-26). And if Sarah is our mother, then as the seeds of Sarah, no matter the challenge; we should give birth to the living like our mother gave birth to all living. We must harness the blessing of Sarah, the mother of all living, to become mothers and fathers of living children. By the Spirit of the Most High, you shall not give birth to a still born nor suffer any miscarriage any more in the name of Jesus Christ.

Come along with me to the next chapter and see how it is that God has a stake in the children you are about to bear.

# Scriptural Notes

- Genesis 1: 21-22, 27-28

- Genesis 2: 7

- Genesis 3: 15-17, 20

- Genesis 25: 21-23; 30: 22-24

- Exodus 1: 7-12; 23:25

- Leviticus 25: 20-21

- Numbers 5: 11-28

- Deuteronomy 7: 14

- Deuteronomy 23: 5

- Judges 13: 2-5

- Nehemiah 13: 2

- Job 1: 10-12; 2:6; 14:4

- Psalm 22: 9-10

- Psalm 71: 6

- Psalm 81: 16

- Psalm 147: 13

- Isaiah 11: 6

- Isaiah 27: 3-4, 6;

- Isaiah 51: 2; 66:9

- Isaiah 65: 23

- Jeremiah 23: 28; 33:6

- Jeremiah 29: 11

- Hosea 9: 11, 14

- Mathew 3:9

- Mathew 13: 24-30; 27:46, 50-51

- Luke 1: 19-28; 57

- Galatians 4: 22-26

- Revelation 12

# CHAPTER SIX

*God has a Stake in Your Children*

*And I will bless her, and give you a son from her! Yea, I will! bless her, and she shall become a mother of nations; kings of people shall be from her.*

*- Genesis 17:16p*

> *The fact that you are a woman is a proof that you have a womb. Your presence confirms a need on earth*

As we study the lives of people who waited for some time before bearing children, we discover that God has a stake in their producing babies. While God was watching Abraham and Sarah in their barren state, He was arranging how His plan for the earth would be fulfilled through their seed. God determined to display His sovereignty through a nation and thus purposed according to His plan that this nation would be born through Abraham and Sarah at the appointed time. When that appointed (or *right*) time of life came for God to begin preparing to raise the nation, Sarah conceived and bore Isaac. Isaac married Rebekah, and her childbearing was delayed, too, because God was still working out His plan to have two nations. When the right time came for these two nations to be raised, the working of the Spirit of the blessing of the womb was released and she gave birth to two nations.

Likewise, Hannah was also not able to conceive because God had an arrangement to have a prophet named Samuel to instruct the nation Israel that He had created out of Abraham's Seed. In the New Testament, we find Elizabeth waiting for a child because God's plan required a forerunner to go prepare the way of the coming Saviour—John the Baptist, born to Elizabeth at just the right time when the King was about to be born.

## HE WILL SATISFY YOU EARLY WITH HIS GREAT MERCY

Every woman in Bible history whose childbearing was delayed went through that experience to give birth to the fulfillment of God's plan for the nations of the earth. This was what the prophet Isaiah saw when he admonished the barren woman in Isaiah 54 to sing aloud and enlarge her tent for more shall be the children of the woman who has never labored by God's agenda. The category of women described here can be likened to those who have faithfully kept themselves and have been diligent in the Lord's service but have not bore a child. The case of Elizabeth and Zacharias is an example. They were both righteous before God, and perhaps have faithfully kept themselves from their youth. They have also been serving diligently in His service, still without a child (Luke 1:6-8). Women in this category feel sometimes forsaken and denied after waiting for long; but God assures that for such women, He will gather them with His great mercies (Isaiah 54:7-8). It is with His everlasting kindness that He will have mercy on you to conceive your long awaited babies.

His mercy comes into play here. He sees these cases as opportunity to show great mercies to His people, so that many may fear and acknowledge Him as the Most High. Just as He showed great mercies to Elizabeth and Zechariah to be able to conceive; He will show great mercy to you as well. This will happen so that your neighbours and relatives could see that the Lord your God performs His promise of mercy to them that fear Him from generation to generation (Luke 1:50). You shall yet rejoice and people shall come to rejoice with you soon because the Lord is determined, to show His great mercies again to them that fear Him, just as He did to Elizabeth (Luke 1:58) and as reiterated in Isaiah 54:7-8.

Verse 7: "For a small moment have I forsaken thee; but with great mercies will I gather thee".

Verse 8: "In a little wrath I hid my face from thee for a moment; but with everlasting kindness will I have mercy on thee, saith the Lord thy Redeemer".

God is anticipating to show up radically again in this time and season by fulfilling His covenant of mercy to them that fear Him. You will obtain mercy and by His great mercy; you shall bear your seeds regardless. Do not boast about how that you have kept yourself pure from your youth, rather, keep asking for His mercies, and not base your petition on self righteousness!

See what He is saying about you in Isaiah 66:7. He said

concerning you that "before you even travailed, you had brought forth and before you experience birth pain, you were delivered of a man child". This implies that according to the pattern of things in the heavens, you have already brought forth. His perception about your case is that you are already with children. It may seem ridiculous to say this about you; but it is so, that you might manifest the miraculous according to His strange acts. His integrity is therefore committed to ensure that you experience that such thing which no one has heard of. He shall cause you to conceive and bring forth in the flesh by His mighty power through His great mercies upon you.

## THAT ALL MAY CONSIDER AND KNOW HE IS

God has a stake in bringing to earth your children because this is one of the ways that people may know, consider, and acknowledge that He is great in counsel and mighty in deeds. The way of the Spirit of conception is higher than our ways and by this act, He is the miracle working God. His works are past finding out and if no one truly knows how bones do grow in the womb of her that is with child (Ecclesiastes 11:5); therefore, you must not doubt His ability to make all things grow in your womb for your baby's formation. He is more than able to form a baby in your womb. For out of you shall yet proceed thanksgiving, and the voice of them that make merry (babies), because the Lord your God will multiply you and you shall not be few, and will also glorify you, and you shall not be small (Jeremiah 30: 19).

He will be faithful to His word to multiply you. He has done this before and can do it again and again. In the beginning, after creation, when God wanted men to multiply on the face on the earth (Genesis 6:1), according to His laid down plan, He made sure that it happened despite the curse. From Adam's lineage, the first man, to that of Noah's, it was recorded that, sons and daughters, and sons respectively, were born to them all. This is the main theme of Genesis 5. According to this chapter: after He created them male and female (verse 2), a chain of family lineages was reproduced to bring about the multiplication of men on earth according to God's plan. We were told Adam begat Seth (verse 3); Seth begat Enos (verse 6); Enos begat Cainan (verse 9); Cainan begat Mahalaleel (verse 12);Mahalaleel begat Jared (verse 15); Jared begat Enoch (verse 18); Enoch begat Methuselah (verse 21); Methuselah begat Lamech (verse 25); Lamech begat Noah (verse 28); and Noah begat Shem, Ham, and Japheth. Each of them, gave birth to sons and daughters, apart from Noah with three sons. The chain–Adam–Seth–Enos–Cainan–Mahalaled–Jared–Enoch–Methuselah–Lamech–Noah–led to the event of *when men began to multiply on earth*. The increasing chain in their reproductive cycle made people to multiply on earth. In the ten genealogies, not one was recorded barren. All of them had children!

This is nothing but the act of God and the blessing of God at work to fulfill His laid down plans for the earth. Knowing then that God does not waste His words; I believe these were written and repeated sequentially, for our lessons. There is a blessing coming that shall usher in another divine season of when men began to multiply on the earth. It shall come to pass when sons and daughters shall again be born towards the fulfillment of His purposed plan. It is another era of the baby boom. You know when God wants to do a new thing, He brings it first in view of a revelation before its manifestation.

There is a manifestation of the sons and daughters of God from heaven about to come to earth from these revelations. They are to be for signs and wonders on planet earth to prepare the Lord's people for His coming.

## YOUR SEED WILL EXECUTE HIS FUTURE PLANS

Dear one, know that there is a plan and an agenda that God wants executed on earth before the world ends, and He will accomplish it through people who have not been corrupted by the existing world system. He actually needs your kind to raise this breed of children. He is raising Seeds who will bruise the head of Satan and his cohorts in these last days. These Seeds are not ordinary Seeds! They are uncommon breeds! Meanwhile, the devil is afraid to see these Seeds come to the earth because he knows what trouble they will cause him. God, however, is ready to bring these Seeds to the earth through His Spirit in order for His plan to be fulfilled. He has prepared for Himself the Seeds that will declare His generation in these last days according to the prophecy of Isaiah 53:8.

God is raising up children who will usher in the age of the second coming of Jesus Christ. They are a mighty army that will prepare a people ready for the Lord's coming. These are your children spoken about in Joel 2:1-9 that they are the like of whom has never been. In the midst of this worldly gloominess and end time mood, these children still shall emerge great and strong. Aren't you blessed to have your children to come as part of these children described here in Joel 2?

This kind of children is conceived only by the Spirit of God Himself, after the workings of the Spirit and not after the workings of the flesh. When His Spirit is required for conception to take place, it indicates that the Seed is an instrument for His glory, which means He is committed to bring the Seed to life. So God has a stake in the children you will bear, and that is why you are relying on His life-giving Spirit to put life in your womb. The Bible refers to these children as the heritage of the Lord (God's property, meaning God's future) and says that they are like arrows in the hand of a warrior according to Psalm 127:3-4. In this case God is the Chief Warrior; the mighty man of valour, and the man of war is His name. Heritage means inheritance, so these children are the inheritance that God is using to face the enemy at the gate from one generation to another. He will mount these Seeds with authority to quench the fiery darts of their enemies and humble wickedness before good. Happy is He, too, when He has His quiver full of them to face His enemies at the gate. That's why I know He wants them here more than you do.

Moreover, He is dedicated to His reward plan for those who serve Him and wait for Him. Since part of His reward program is the fruit of the womb, and He has sworn by His holiness that He will not lie to us, then, He will perform His reward programme to you who serves and wait for Him. Exodus 23:25-26 highlights the catalogue of things in His reward programme. This is nothing less than the blessing of Sarah, the fruit of the womb, and is a surety for those who serve Him. You are guaranteed a reward of service by God, and being a stakeholder in your fruitfulness, He will redeem His reward program to you.

*His praise is in the mouth of those children you shall soon bear*

## HIS PRAISE IS ON THE LIPS OF YOUR BABIES

As a matter of fact, so long as the

earth remain, people must praise Him from generation to generation. As a result, as one generation is passing away, another generation is created to praise Him (Psalm 78:4). His praise is in the mouth of those children you shall soon bear. Your children are God's inheritance whose praise is on their lips, and for that reason, they must come to the earth to sing those praises on their lips to God. David emphasized this, teaching us why God has a stake in the children you are about to bear–because they are God's strength to defeat the enemies of God and avenge the righteous (Psalm 8:2). David saw that "out of the mouth of babes and nursing infants God has ordained strength, because of His enemies, that He may silence the enemy and the avenger," and that is why David went further to say that for this reason God is mindful of man, always thinking of making man who will have dominion over His works.

Somewhere in Hosea 14:8, God emphasized to the seeds of Abraham (Israelites) that their fruit is found in Him, hence, they had better returned to Him. Any fruit of the body or of the land is found in Him and in nothing else.

> ➤ Abraham understood that God has a stake in the son he bore and so when it was time to get Isaac a wife, he assigned his oldest servant to undertake this task and did not send him out without an accompanied blessing to enable him prosper on this search (Genesis 24:2-7). He could see that through Isaac, God's plans would be executed.

> ➤ The same was with Isaac too when he grew old. He has been made to understand over time that God has a stake in his children; hence, going by the account in Genesis 27, he longed

earnestly to pronounce the blessing before his death.

➤ Isaac's seeds also understood well the efficacy of the blessing to the extent that Jacob was ready to deceive (while his mother was ready to take his curse upon herself in case he was found out) and Esau was even ready to commit murder for the blessing. This family lineage knows the worth of the blessing, that it is tantamount to God been committed to change the status of the blessed.

➤ And Jacob, also at old age did pronounce the blessing upon his children (Genesis 49) because he could recognize that the God of his fathers had a stake in his children.

## HE CALLS THEM ALREADY BLESSED

How much more God's pronouncements of blessing and the effecting of increase on His own people, are available to us today because He has a claim on the fruits of our body. In some cases in the Bible, God was pronouncing His blessing on the offspring of the children of Israel (Isaiah 44:3b & Deuteronomy 7:13a) and even calls the unborn produce of their bodies blessed. These are children yet to be born but He already calls them blessed (Deuteronomy 28:4a). And if He already blessed them, then He will see to it He brings them onto planet earth to exhibit the blessings.

Verse 3b: "...I will pour my spirit upon thy seed and my blessing upon thine offspring"

Verse 13a: "And He will love thee, and bless thee, and multiply thee: He will also bless the fruit of thy womb ..."

Verse 4a: "Blessed shall be the fruit of thy body ..."

Your children are one of those God is mindful of creating on earth to dominate according to His plan so He calls them blessed. These children about to be born are part of those God will use to silence His enemies. These children are the ones whom the Lord Himself will train in the ways of righteous war. As they are taught of God Himself by the working of His Spirit, these children will become mighty warriors and God's weapon to defeat His enemies on the earth. They will have His word always in their mouths, and when they speak His word, it will run swiftly to perform the given tasks. Eyes have not seen this kind of children before. They are the ones who will bring hope to the hopeless nations and restore the foundations of shaky economies.

*He knows that a house is required in the body to breed a baby so He fashioned the woman with a womb*

They are wonderful children! The children you will bear will represent the interest of His Kingdom on earth, the interest of your country, and the interest of the world. They are kings who will govern their respective countries with justice, fairness, and equity amidst prevailing injustice and inequality in the world. They will tolerate no friendship with poverty in their respective countries nor condone insecurity of lives and properties. These are active and selfless ones who will be committed to give hope again to the widows, orphans, and helpless. Are you not blessed that these are the features of the children you have been expecting? They shall speak with you soon because they have also to speak to the enemies of God at the gate, so they will no longer tarry.

Examining the history of expectant mothers in the Bible has provided us with proof positive that your own long-awaited Seed shall be mighty on the earth and, because this is in God's plan, they will become the reality of your lives. Your Seed will take the baton from older generations to lift high His flag from one generation to another. If you are Christ's, then your children are the succeeding generations who will lift up His banner in their own dispensation. They will proclaim his love and power on earth and turn the hearts of wicked men and women to God, preparing for the Lord a people ready for His coming. God has a stake in those Seeds; your children are privileged. Your grandchildren and great grandchildren are God's inheritance who will offer the sacrifices of praise with their anointed lips. Because He requires your Seed to spread the gospel in their own time, He will bring them to life here on earth and not just in His heavenly plan. Just as Isaac was from Heaven to Earth, so shall your children come to earth for He has declared them in Heaven as already blessed.

They are God's prophecies who have gone forth and would become flesh and live among men on planet earth. God does not speak empty words. He does not say what He cannot do nor declare what He does not mean. If He has already spoken to you in several prophecies through His word how your children have a role in bringing His plan to pass, then simply believe that you will have those children. Because God's prophecies are with you, His Spirit is committed to work them out to prove His integrity! Your children are part of the disciples, apostles, evangelists, teachers and preachers, and givers in the market places that God yearns to reach. He needs prophets and at the same time you need sons: hence an exchange must take place. Your daughters about to come are part of the prophetesses God needs to fulfill His plans on earth. Be conscious of this and you shall soon carry God's promise in the flesh. Therefore rejoice wear the carriage of the kings' mother and kings' father because God has a stake in your coming Seed.

## YOUR WOMB: A HOUSE CREATED TO BREED HIS SEEDS

What's more, God designed you with a womb so that you can carry children with it and you know He does not waste His resources. He does not create what would not be useful to Him nor to humanity. He knows that a house is required in the body to breed a baby so He fashioned the woman with a womb with which to breed His Seeds. If that was not a useful part, He would not have created a womb in the woman's body in the first place. But because God knows what He was doing and in that He is upright, He made a house in women for children to grow. If a human being will not just build a house on earth for the sake of building one, not to be inhabited; then God will not give you a womb that will not be inhabited by His Seeds. Hence, because your womb has been designed and constructed to carry children, you must carry children with your womb since for this purpose it was created.

The fact that you are a woman is a proof that you have a womb. Your presence confirms a need on earth. Your womb is like a house fashioned to nurture His Seeds to a maturity level, where life enters. God is a builder, human estate developer, owner; you are the housing estate developed; while your baby is the resident of the finished building. His desire is for your womb to house His tenant. Your Seeds are His Seeds so why worry; He wants them here more than you do, and therefore He is at work to see they come through your womb. God can only accomplish this desire on earth through humans with a womb, and you are His only hope of bringing forth these promised children, so relax! Above all, if God could have a son, His only begotten Son, then you will have a son too at least. So be glad! For you shall conceive His inheritance soon.

# Scriptural Notes

- Genesis 5: 1-32; 6: 1

- Genesis 24: 2-7

- Genesis 27: 1-4

- Genesis 49: 1-27

- Exodus 23: 25-26

- Deuteronomy 7: 13a

- Deuteronomy 28: 4a

- Psalm 8: 2

- Psalm 78: 4

- Psalm 127: 3-4

- Ecclesiastes 11:5

- Isaiah 44: 3b

- Isaiah 53: 8

- Isaiah 54: 1-3; 7-8

- Isaiah 66: 7-9

- Hosea 14: 8

- Joel 2: 1-9

- Luke 1:6-8

- Luke 1:50, 58

# CHAPTER SEVEN
*Expect Attacks on Your Confidence*

*And I will bless her, and give you a son from her! Yea, I will bless her, and she shall become a mother of nations; kings of people shall be from her*

*- Genesis 17:16p*

*There is a blessing coming and you need to prepare for it*

You might be wondering, *If God is indeed a stakeholder why am I childless?* It is very likely that this thought will run through your mind, but I implore you to shut it out. As an expectant mother that is not the kind of thought you should entertain because you do not want to be in the position of contesting that you shall bear your own children. You know in your heart that you will surely conceive, just as you know that you are a female and nothing can be done to change your status to a male.

The state of your thought life regarding this issue is imperative for your conception to take place. This is because your thinking and your prayer has equal acceptance before God. Thoughts have equivalent access to God as prayers do; going by Ephesians 3:20. According to this Epistle, God perceives our thoughts and prayers as same, with an equal opportunity of receiving answers as He is able to do above all that we ask or think. By this, I am sure you cannot afford to be the one nullifying your prayers with your unstable thoughts of perhaps that you may not bear. The two must align for a manifestation to happen.

You must know, however, that when you embark on this provocative walk of faith you will be rigorously scrutinized. You will be subject to attacks on your faith and the confidence you are building that you shall bear a child. These attacks will be initiated by the enemy of your Seed (the devil) but perpetuated through people. The people he will use are usually those who are close to you. They will come with worldly advice. They might suggest that you consider divorcing so you can marry another wife or husband. They may advise you to consider adoption and forget about still conceiving yours. Some may even counsel you to consult foreign gods. Some will hurl abuse, humiliation, and insults at you and may even withdraw friendship from you.

Listen: This is normal for you who are to become a king's mother. Their humiliation, insults, abuses, and mockery that you have not borne is actually part of offered prayers to speedily bring about a manifestation of your long awaited miracle. They are helping you to serve God a reminder notice so that you can be remembered on this matter of conceiving a seed. So know that their mockery is working together for your change of status; because they are part of the aiding tools to bring about your season of miracle.

There will be attempts to distract you from the faith walk and divert your attention from what will work out for you eventually to what will not work. Remember Job, beset with all those calamities, whose own wife came to attack his confidence and prescribed that he curse God while his friends reminded him how much he must have sinned against God to cause all that grief. God kept quiet and was watching everyone, especially the attitude and actions of Job to see if he would lose focus. And what happened to Job eventually? God blessed him because he was found not to cast off restraint despite his predicament. Even though his own wife and friends could not envision his comeback, Job himself did not yield to their bad advice and pressure.

*God perceives our thoughts and prayers as same, with an equal opportunity of receiving answers*

As an expectant mother you cannot afford to give in to external pressures and attacks on your confidence. If you do, you will be the one to lose out at the end of the day. There is a blessing coming and you need to prepare for it. You have to be conscious that you are carrying a precious Seed that is not visible to the ordinary eye yet is as real as your flesh. When those arrows come to pierce your confidence, shield them with the word of life that is laid up in your heart and act on it. As a mother who shall soon bear, your confidence on this matter will be rewarded so you cannot afford to waver. Rather, bolster your faith and confidence by filling yourself with the Word of God assuring you of your conception and the promises of your Seed unborn. These living promises in you will always rise above idle talk and useless worldly counsel from those who, though they care for you, just don't understand the workings of the blessing.

I know it might be a bit difficult and tense, especially when in-laws are involved, but please do not allow their pressure to burst the confidence that you have been building with blocks of the words of faith. Do not allow their pressure to squeeze out what you have been labouring to build by pondering night and day on their words of worry and concern. You cannot afford to misuse your energy in this way because you are nearer to your salvation than ever, and every step in the faith walk counts. Use your energy instead to meditate on the fact that you have received strength to conceive and that the Spirit of the blessing of Sarah is working on you and you cannot afford to grieve the Spirit with negative emotions.

Thank them with warm gratitude for their concern when they remind you that you are yet to bear and show them the look of a blessed mother of children, which you are indeed. Do not frown or show a sad countenance when they come to you with great concern. You are not who they see you to be. You are who God sees you to be, a fruitful womb with children. Don't allow their sayings to affect your mood. Train yourself in the Word and build up confidence based on these words of the Spirit till it becomes obvious that you are not beaten. Don't give any indication that you are beaten or that you are down. Rejoice, for that is what the word of faith and confidence asks you to do in Isaiah 54. God is waiting to commend your habitual singing and attitude of rejoicing and the fact that you have not been moved thus far.

God knows it if you are feeling beaten and down, He can see your heart, so step up your confidence because you are giving birth after the workings of the Spirit of the blessing of Sarah upon your life. I know it can be hard, too, when friends invite you to the naming ceremony of their children and you feel a little shame, but take heart because you can choose to rest in your confidence that you will be inviting them to your own child's naming ceremony before long. Dance with them and rejoice at such occasions. Be sure to carry the baby before you leave there and dance with him or her if permitted, because you will also carry your own soon. Your faith and confidence in God is paramount when you want the working of the Spirit of the blessing of Sarah to continue working on you. Avoid going out there and acting as though the blessing of Sarah is not working upon you. It is working on you at all times so remain conscious of this working in order not to act contrary.

Do not forget that without faith it is impossible to please God. It is like taking the tablets prescribed by a medical doctor in order to become well if you are sick. The doctor instructs his patient how to use the medication and when to use it and even warns the patient of the danger of discontinued or inconsistent usage. The doctor always warns that the drug will only achieve the desired result if taken in the manner prescribed. Thus, the patient takes the drug as the doctor prescribed; following the instruction judiciously in faith that doing so will make him well. That is exactly how it is with the greatest Physician. As a matter of fact, the earthly doctors learned this technique from Him.

When the blessing of Sarah is working on you, you cannot afford to abort it with your tongue or with your sad countenance, for then He will go away. What comes out from your tongue during this waiting time is formidable and so you could use it to form life and not death. Remember the Words of Jesus in Mathew 12:37 that "for by your words you will be justified and by your word you will be condemned." Just like the children of Israel judged themselves by asking "Can God? Can God? Can God?" and provoked judgement upon themselves (Psalm 78: 19- 22) by doubting His wonder working power having experienced His mighty deeds. A people who have lived with a repetitive display of God's power could still possess a feeling of uncertainty about the authenticity of this power. There is tendency that a waiting mother could act likewise. Having tasted of the power of the highest in her career, finances business, ministry, and marriage; she could still be apprehensive about giving birth to her own Seeds. Our actions, words, thoughts and meditations must not reflect apprehensions or distrust in His power to bring His promises to pass.

Let words of faith be found in your mouth night and day as your proofs for justification while the accuser of the brethren is busy accusing you day and night, too, before the father. The father should see reasons to justify your becoming a mother and give no room for your condemnation. It is possible to speak positively on a daily basis even if it means practicing it until it becomes your mother tongue. No matter how tormented you are as a result of still waiting, the express statement that should proceed out of your mouth is, "It is well with my Soul" or scream, "I am blessed! I am blessed! I am blessed! I am blessed! And I know I am blessed!!!!!!!". Speak blessings because those who love blessing shall eat of its fruits.

Know that your tongue is a powerful being. The tongue can invoke and revoke, depending on how you use it, so do not stop making decrees and pronouncements. The tongue is that part of God that pronounces the blessing upon His people. Even when He curses them due to their disobedience, He turns around and equally pronounces a higher blessing to override the curses when they repent. Thus, you knowing that your descendant shall be many; your offspring like the grass of the earth and you shall fill the face of the world with fruit (Job 5:25 & Isaiah 27:6); this awareness should live with you. You should release pronouncements of blessing of the breast and of the womb on yourself with your tongue and the great man in your life should equally join you in doing so. There should be no room for contrary pronouncements around you regarding your fruitfulness.

Provide an inviting atmosphere for the working of the Spirit of the womb by being conscious of its working on you and living it out. Do not engage the workings of the Spirit of Sarah today and do petty things tomorrow to show them in heaven that you believe otherwise. It will not work that way. Take the complete dose by eating the Word, speaking the Word, and acting upon the Word of your promised Seeds. When you see a woman or a man wearing an all-white outfit, check him out for that period and see how careful he is, being conscious of the white garment, to avoid unnecessary stains. That is how you are as a king's mother-to-be.

Remember that God sees the heart and is a discerner of the

thoughts and intents of the heart before they are acted out (Hebrews 4: 12). He alone can see if you still doubt the possibility of giving birth to your own children. He can see your thoughts if you are still exercising fear and panicking that perhaps you will exit the earth without carrying your own child. These thoughts trouble the hearts of some people whose hearts are not properly guarded. The devil gets excited when you are thinking like this, or worrying that you will not bear till death, which is impossible with the working of the blessing on your life. When the words of the blessing of Sarah are released upon you, they run swiftly towards you since they have been sent out to accomplish a purpose, but on getting to the destination, the heart is repulsive. The words of blessing meet with several thoughts that are contrary to the workings of the Spirit of the blessing of the womb and thus are rendered inactive. You need to sweep out your heart thoroughly on a daily basis because you do not know the day of your release.

You have to fight the good fight of faith to keep your heart in a condition conducive for the working of the blessing of the womb to alight and do a quick work on you. The Apostle Paul foresaw that many of us would face challenges in getting our thoughts to align with the Word of God, which is the Spirit of God, and quickly told us about his own ordeal (Romans 7:15-25). He explained to us in detail how he acted contrary to what the Word expected from him and exclaimed that nothing good dwelled in him and how there was a warring against his mind trying to bring him into captivity that eventually succeeded at making him a wretched man that God did not want him to be.

He tells us, however, how we can avoid such a situation in our own lives through Christ Jesus, who is the spoken Word of God. Paul did not stop there because he knew how stubborn the negative thoughts warring against our mind can be. So he went further and emphasized again the enormity of the work we need to do to ensure that we always win the battle of the mind (2 Corinthians 10:4-7). He advised that we should be conscious of the extent of the working of the mighty power at our disposal in Christ Jesus in pulling down strongholds in thoughts, in words, in deeds, and those already resident in our minds. He referred to them as high things in 2 Corinthians 10:5. When the thoughts of in-laws creep into your heart they have a way of dominating major thoughts in the heart and become the high thing on the platform of the heart for the day and even at night. God can see these thoughts on your thought priority list. They do not please God because they are devoid of faith. The Apostle Paul also emphasized to us how obstinate these thoughts can be and declared them to be a *high thing* that exalts itself. The nature of these negative thoughts is to seek governance, so that once we entertain them they rise in our heart until they are exalted over all other beliefs in that system.

Thus Paul went further and advised us that we should not entertain them in the first place! As soon as you see them coming, quickly cast them down, bring them down. It is like spotting a cockroach on your wall inside the kitchen about to come down into your pot of soup. You do not watch it crawl down and spoil your lunch, do you? You hit it hard immediately and bring it down yourself into the trash bin before it dominates your kitchen and messes up the whole place. It is the same with rats. If we do not tolerate these minor destructive agents in our kitchens, why on earth would we entertain the major destructive agents in our cooking hearts that guide the issues of life?

Paul advises that we do not sit idly by and let them drive us into wretchedness but rather quickly cast them down and give no room for the devil in our thoughts in the first place. Before he exalts his throne in your heart, cast him down. And for you to cast him down, you must have the necessary weapons to finish those thoughts at hand for there's no time in the heat of thought–battle for scrambling for your weapons. The same way you always have something readily available in your kitchen to bring down any little insect you spot on your wall, so you should have the Word of Life readily available to dispel the lies the devil is trying to sell you. This means that you must be fully armed with the Word of God. Drink it like water and eat it like food.

Be ready always with whatever it is you know will help you gain an upper hand over negative thoughts, and be armed with the truth. If it is to play messages in your car at every slightest move you make, do it! If it is to play inspiring worship songs to keep your soul alive, please do it! If what works more for you is to pray for as long as you can to have Spirit-filled imaginations, please do it! If interceding for others and praying in the Holy Ghost works for you, embrace it! Go out and spend time with your loved ones who inspire you spiritually and ignite your flame. Attend mid-week services at church and dance during the praise and worship like you have never danced before. Take some time out as often as you can to confess aloud all the words of the blessing of Sarah, using your mouth to recreate your mood and a conducive environment for the miracle you have been expecting.

Just do all you can to get those evil and negative thoughts filtered away from your heart. For there must be no hangover noticed around the corridors of your heart. It must all be swept out thoroughly and neatly, too, for the working of the Spirit of the blessing of Sarah to have a free hand. God will reward this in you as well, so do not entertain any negative thought for a second even when the poser comes from your household; rather let it go, for it is not new under the sun. There is nothing wrong with you, believe it! You are good as God called you good in the beginning. All you need is the blessing of the womb and in the name of Jesus Christ, the Spirit of the Highest will come upon you to work out the blessing of Sarah; and you shall speak with your children as He has promised you.

I have learned to build up my confidence in God despite what people around me think of the situation at hand. Thus I end up never being ashamed in any way. Today, I am always grateful to God for teaching me early on how to build up confidence in Him, and trust me when I tell you that it pays a lot to do so. I had to learn how to engage this vital weapon when I noticed from experience that the older I got and the more I attained, the tougher were the challenges that came along. And knowing that there are yet greater heights to be reached, I requested help from the Holy Spirit to build my confidence and trust in His Word. I have reaped great rewards as a result; it has worked out great benefits for me and I believe it will work out even greater benefits for you. So build up your most holy faith as well as your confidence which attracts great reward.

Do not allow even the misbehavior of your spouse to make you lose your confidence of conceiving your own children. This is because if Satan cannot get external bodies to attack your faith, he will use your flesh (that is your spouse or use you against yourself). Do not allow him access through any means, not even you the expectant one. At this juncture, I want to address the issue of spouses misbehaving to each other as a result of weariness in waiting for their miracle children as brought to my knowledge by His Spirit. I once attended a prophetic prayer meeting where the Holy Spirit particularly picked on a woman who had been waiting to conceive for nine years.

According to the charges against her, she has been insubordinate to her husband, abusive, intolerable, and has suddenly lost words seasoned with grace in her mouth–all as a result of waiting. The husband being a Christian would sometimes keep quiet while at other times he would reciprocate until this day when the Holy Spirit exposed her anomalies at the meeting. The Holy Spirit emphasized that she (especially) and her husband have been the ones prolonging her conception because of these unacceptable attitudes toward each other. She was advised of the need to change her ways before she could attract the Spirit which can put life in her womb. The reason given was that He cannot work in a place where there is strive, insubordination, and frequent use of unfriendly languages, and so she has been responsible for keeping their presence away all along. Then immediately, she broke down in tears and asked God for mercy. Five months after this incident, I saw her again. And at this time, to my amazement she was already four months pregnant, and looking radiant with joy.

On this day, I realized for the first time that God does not joke with spouses fulfilling their obligations to one another and acting accordingly in love and submissiveness towards each other. Husband and wife expecting to conceive a blessing such as a baby should not be fighting each other because the blessing will not come. Though we might think all these things do not really matter but each matters to those who will work out a living being in you and considering they have a stake in the child's upbringing too. The One who will leave behind a blessing for you on His visit to your home must meet you prepared for it. That is why we were told in Psalm 133 that it is good for us to dwell together in unity because there the Lord commanded the blessing and life. What you are looking for is a blessing and life; and the One who commands it to earth have required that you walk in unity with those around you. This lesson teaches husbands and wives not to give room to friction in any form as God will only honour your unity of spirit, obedience to His Word, and confidence in Him that He will do it though it tarries.

*Top up your confidence daily, consistently recharge it and raise it even higher day by day because you will need it to prevail*

Therefore, top up your confidence daily, consistently recharge it, and raise it even higher day by day because you will need it to prevail. With it, the Spirit of the blessing of Sarah and even the blessing of Abraham will always be with you. Your faith will attract and retain the blessing. Above all, the mercy of God will speak over your life, and you will be highly favoured by His Spirit in the name of Jesus Christ. Hence, start behaving as the blessed among women because that is what the blessing is working out in your life. Believe this reality as your end result-that, after all, you will become a mother of children and a father of children.

Human frailties can deflate our hope and confidence and lead us to focus more on the seeming impossibilities and shortcomings than on the promise. But the persistence of faith, together with moments of belief with no doubts, will take you to your long- awaited destination. Allow the intake of the Word to stretch your human capacity to imagine beyond the reality of your present situation. These advises are the foolishness of God and it is better to learn His foolishness than embrace the contemporary wisdom of men. Remember that the foolishness of God (1Corinthians 1:25) is wiser than the wisest of the wisdom of men, so stay with His foolishness to see His power in display in your case. As you do these, that bit of your humanity is constantly fed by His Spirit and you shall see your children surround you because the blessing of Sarah would work in you.

You are the winner in this matter. God's children are destined to win, so, the enemy is only working for God again in your case. We could see from the story of Job how that Satan has been using his time working tirelessly for God. I believe that all his running to and fro the earth, and hurling afflictions at women are invariably for the promotion of the workings of God on earth–the Supreme One. Even at times when it seems the devil is winning or having a fun-fair with his schemes and operational strategies, you will soon realise that he did not win anyway. The conclusion of the whole matter is always that he has spent all his time and efforts working altogether for God's glory and for your good.

Even if you were told that yours is a problem or condition that is hereditary or generational, through the working of the blessing

# Scriptural Notes

- Job 5: 25

- Psalm 78: 19-22

- Psalm 133

- Isaiah 27: 6

- Isaiah 54: 1-3

- Mathew 12:37

- Romans 7: 15-25

- I Corinthians 1: 25

- 2 Corinthians 10: 4-7

- Ephesians 3: 20

- Hebrews 4: 12

# CHAPTER EIGHT

*Barrenness Shall Soon Loose You*

*And I will bless her, and give you a son from her! Yea will bless her, and she shall*

*become a mother of nations; kings of people shall be from her*

*- Genesis 17:16p*

| |
|---|
| *You are different, and you will give birth* |

**B**arrenness shall soon loose you. If you can make it a habit to live according to the prophecy of Isaiah 54, then you will be surprised how quickly your children shall soon occupy your table. Barrenness will loose you completely and be gone without a trace. Though the enemy we contend with (the devil) can be very stubborn and does not always want to lie low, know this: He cannot stand the presence of the Lion of the tribe of Judah working in you, and thus he will soon loose you completely. You are more than a conqueror and in Christ Jesus an overcomer in this world. And thus you will overcome barrenness. Hold on to God because barrenness is about to loose its grip over you. The working of the blessing of the womb is a work after the Spirit of God and the work culminates in life. The life is the life of the children that you have waited for so long.

What you are looking for is the creation of life, and it is like that can beget like. It is the life of God that gives life, and life is what you want to give birth to. The life is in the Word of God and it is the Spirit of life in Christ Jesus that makes free. When His Word dwells in you, nothing will be able to withstand you, including barrenness. In other words, the fullness of the indwelling Word can impregnate you so that you will begin to give birth to sons and daughters and then barrenness will eventually loose you. The wonder-working Spirit in the Word will move upon you and in you, breaking every curse of barrenness until it looses you completely.

Act on Isaiah 54. Do the setting of your house as though you have children. Do not say, "I do not have children yet, so we do not need a family dining table." Set up that table and surround it with the number of chairs you will need for however many children you want under your roof. Decorate their bedrooms and purchase their clothing. Name them before their arrival and call their names as though they are already under the same roof with you. Give their own offerings in church services as though they were there with you in church giving their own offering to God as well. Remember the blessing of Malachi 3: 10 when you pay tithes and offerings, how He would pour out on you such a blessing that a room cannot contain! Test Him in this on the behalf of your expected children and see if you will not need more rooms to contain their arrivals.

Children are part of this blessing which we will not have room enough to contain and this blessing will be the certainty of your life. Keep at it, for the vision (your children) is for an appointed time, though it tarries, wait for it, and it shall speak in the end (Habakkuk 2:3). Even after much bad seasons of weariness on this matter, there is hope for you. And even at the end of that long rope called patience, there is still hope for you. There is hope still in the midst of this much holding-on. The Pharaohs of this world (fibroid, tumors, miscarriages, etc.) might contend with your conception, nonetheless, your expectation shall not be cut short. You will eventually hear your children speak to you. They shall speak at the end of your waiting and not only to you but also to the enemies at the gate. This was what Abraham did not know when he agreed to go unto Sarah's handmaid. The fact that Isaac will speak with him in his lifetime after all became the actuality of his and Sarah's life. Abraham's lack of understanding that he would one day speak to his son led him astray.

Whenever I log onto the Winners website, I see a series of couples giving testimonies with their babies in hand as undeniable proof, to the working of the blessing of Sarah. These traced cases on the working of the blessing of the womb will help to bolster your faith and you shall become liberated by the words of these testimonies. I have decided to document some of these testimonies in the pages that follow to encourage you and strengthen your faith and make barrenness loose its hold completely on you. These testimonies and others from ministries whose leaders are committed to the pronouncement of the blessing will challenge you to stand up, wipe the tears off your face, and engage the Spirit of the blessing of Sarah in your own case as well. It requires a conscious effort, and this is what characterizes all of these testifiers. They believed they were not barren, and their Prophets and Pastors did continuously pronounce the blessing of conception on them; so today they cannot be labelled barren for they all have a change of story like Sarah, the mother of all living.

## Testimonies from Faith Tabernacle
Date: 02/03/08
Names: Prince & Mrs. A. Samuel
Duration: 20 years of waiting ended

This couple had been without a child for the past 20 years but they believed that they would carry their own children and so they did not stop following God. According to their testimony, they go to Shiloh (An annual gathering of members of Living Faith Church from all over the world) every year tendering their petition to God to bring His promises to pass in their lives. They attended Shiloh six times with no result, but they were not discouraged. They were both sure that they would conceive their own children. During the seventh Shiloh they attended, they went believing that seven signifies perfection and completion and engaged the Spirit of the blessing of the Womb through Dr. David Oyedepo's books on this issue and his teachings. Then the working of the Spirit of the blessing of Sarah perfected its work on them and by February 2007, the woman conceived and gave birth to Miracle in November 2007. **Note here that this couple never thought that they would not bear.** They were so sure their Seed will speak to them, though it may tarry, that they kept going to Shiloh, year in and year out, building up their faith and confidence through books and teachings on this subject, and today they are speaking to their baby.

Date: 13/12/07
Name: Mrs. Favour O.
Duration: 13 years of waiting

This woman's case is incredible but true. In 2001 she was diagnosed of cancer of the cervix and was told that she would die if she did not have her uterus, cervix, and womb removed. The doctor also told her that this procedure would end her chances of conceiving. Later that same year, she had the life-saving surgery that removed virtually all of her reproductive organs, thus making it factually impossible for her to conceive. **This faithful woman, however, decided to approach God on this matter and insisted that despite all these odds she must carry her own baby in her lifetime.** She recognized that God is the maker of all living beings and can thus create and recreate at will, and so she kept coming to Shiloh and listening to the teachings of Dr. David Oyedepo. In one of his teachings, she heard him proclaim that "there is hope of a tree, if it be cut down, that it will sprout again, and that the tender branch thereof will not cease" (Job 14:7). **Then she recognized that this word was referring to her and she believed her womb would grow again** and that she had come to Shiloh to be blessed with a new womb since the old one had been cut down. After Shiloh 2005, she conceived after the working of the Spirit and precisely before Shiloh 2006, she delivered of a bouncing baby boy named *Emmanuel*. Her testimony is phenomenal and there is no explanation for it except God's blessing for fruitfulness. Medical science cannot afford to comprehend such unusual acts, which confound all medical knowledge and practice. Did you notice that this woman was attentive enough to identify the very Word that addresses her case during the sermons at the event? She did not go there as a spectator, she went to gather her own *'Word-team member'* with which to fight and win her case against barrenness. There are scriptures addressing your case; be alert enough to identify and gather them when you are listening to sermons or searching through the Word. They are your armoury; there lies your weapons of mass destruction against barrenness. Therefore, even if you do not have a womb, do not write yourself off because you have what it takes to overcome.

Date: 12/12/07
Name: Mrs. Aderonke O.
Duration: 11 years of waiting

This woman lost her first baby in 1995 and had been unable to conceive another since then. Her search for fertility led her to travel to eastern Europe to undergo a fertilization transfer that was very expensive and was to no avail. **On account of her inability to conceive she was called names, such as "cow's mother" and "pawpaw's enemy," but she believed that her story would change.** At last she resorted to God and continued serving faithfully as a sanctuary keeper in the Winners Chapel Otta. One day, as she had just finished discharging her sanctuary keeper duties, she heard the Bishop teaching, saying lie down wherever you are on the ground and request from the God of heaven anything you have desired. So she obeyed and requested that she would conceive her own baby. She poured out her heart to God in her dialect while on the ground and said, "O Lord, if truly you called this your servant, let me carry my own baby in my womb and on my back so I can testify to this truth that you have indeed sent your servant." Then in 2006, she noticed her belly was protruding and went to see her doctor. He examined her and concluded that her case had gone from bad to worse because she now had diabetes, which explained why her abdomen was protruding. She left his office still believing God for her conception and after six months she noticed her stomach was protruding so conspicuously now it could not be hidden. Then she went back to her doctor for a re-check because she did not believe the diabetes was causing her latest protrusion. After examining her, her doctor started to apologize because she did not have diabetes at all but a baby in her womb, and so at the end of her nine-month term she had a baby boy named *David*. Whose report will you believe to have your long awaited children? The report of the Lord cannot fail you.

Date: 30/03/08
Name: Mrs. Ayeni I.
Duration: 12 years of waiting ended

This woman's testimony is amazing. Her faith was superb in the sense that she never once gave up. She succeeded in making barrenness loose its grip on her through her continuous giving and intensified service in church as a sanctuary keeper with the mind that she would be rewarded someday if she did not faint. According to her testimony, she had been to so many hospitals all to no avail, and when she realised that all doctors' efforts failed, she decided to settle with God who is the Giver and Maker of life.

She lived her life daily with the consciousness that she was a fruitful woman, not a barren woman, through her endless confessions and investing her time in reading books on this topic and studying her Bible. **She bought all her baby's things and went to church with them and even gave offerings on behalf of her unborn baby.** Whenever she saw her monthly cycle, she reminded it that it had to stop flowing because she was expecting a living being and did not want to see it flow as a result. All these she continued to do by faith until she contacted the working of the Spirit of the blessing of the womb and then conceived in 2007 and gave birth to *Samuel.* Barrenness completely loosed her because she was relentless and determined that barrenness would not hold her down forever. This can be your testimony as well!

Date: 13/12/07
Name: Mrs. T. Young
Duration: Over 10 years of waiting

This woman gave birth to triplets after waiting for a child for over 10 years. **She had been to several hospitals seeking a solution to her infertility—all to no reward**. She got fed up with her state and even stopped going to church because, she decided, she could not see the result of her continuous visit to church if she was childless. Then one day, she was told about the Winners Chapel Chapter in Yenegoa, Bayelsa State, where she lives and decided to go and attend the Bible school. She enrolled for the ministry's bible school called {Word Of Faith Bible Institute, WOFBI} classes and afterwards proceeded to attend the advanced Bible classes called the {Leadership Certificate Course, LCC} which ended in August 2006. **She heard the word of life**

**while studying in the Bible classes and became convinced that she was not barren. The words of life got her impregnated** and, with the working of the Spirit of the blessing of the womb, she gave birth in 2007 to a boy whom she named *God's Favour*, a girl named *God's Heritage*, and another girl named *God's Reward*. With the working of the Spirit of the blessing of the womb, the words of life got her impregnated because she had positioned herself for it.

Date: 27/01/08
Name: Mrs. Seyi O.
Duration: 10 years of waiting ended

This woman had been waiting to carry and speak to her own baby for a decade. **She kept coming to church and never gave up on herself because she believed that she was a mother and would deliver her baby.** According to her testimony, she took a further step to see the Dr. David and Faith Oyedepo and they laid hands on her and pronounced upon her the working of the blessing of Sarah, which is the blessing of the womb, and that same month of March in the year 2006, she got impregnated after the Spirit and gave birth to her baby. Today she is speaking to her baby because she forced her way out of the grip of barrenness. Barrenness loosed its grip on her at last because she took conscious steps to attract the working of the blessing of the womb. **The pronouncement of the blessings over us by our spiritual parent is imperative towards attracting our miracles. I believe so much in the blessings of the fathers; it works because it cannot fall to the ground when they are sent by the Most High.** When you believe the words of His prophets no matter how calmly they say it, you shall prosper even in your body.

Names: Mr. & Mrs. A. Francis
Duration: 9 years of waiting

This couple waited for nine years to have their baby. They believed they would bear and did not stop living like it. **They sowed on behalf of their unborn babies,** read books on the subject matter, and today barrenness lost its grip on them after the working of the Spirit of the blessing of the womb as they gave birth to twins. **Note that this couple did not desist from living like they would bear their own children all through the nine years of waiting. They know that the blessing is working already** on their lives because they believed they have been blessed with *all* spiritual blessing in heavenly places as told in Ephesians 1:3. Part of the spiritual blessing from the heavenly places in Christ is the blessing of the womb you are longing for and your request shall be granted you in the name of Jesus Christ.

Date: 27/01/08
Names: Mr. & Mrs. Uche
Duration: 5 years of waiting ended

This couple had waited for five years and had visited doctors who told them that their problem was a case of low sperm count. This couple, however, chose to believe the Word of God that says with God nothing shall be impossible rather than the report of the doctor. They went to church and most times heard Bishop saying that it was their birthright to give birth to their own children, and they held onto these teachings, believing that their right would be given to them, by God. **According to their testimony, they both danced in church as they had never danced before because they were conscious that they would bear,** and in October

2006, the creator of sperm released His Spirit upon the couple and the working of the Spirit of the blessing of the womb enabled the woman to conceive and gave birth to Divine. The grip of barrenness over them was loosed because they consciously provoked upon themselves the working of the Spirit of the blessing of Sarah.

Date: 24/02/08
Names: Mr. & Mrs. Sylvester A.
Duration: 5 years of waiting ending

This couple waited for five years to speak with their children. There is something remarkable about the wife's testimony of how she made her way out of barrenness. **According to her testimony, she danced out at every child dedication in church believing that she was dedicating her own baby alongside with** those whose babies were in their hands for child dedication Whenever she went out with them rejoicing, **she came out with a given name for the baby she had come to dedicate and also** dropped offerings for this baby in faith. **This she continued to do at every child dedication service in church and never wearied of it even when she was not getting an immediate result.** Then one day as she danced out with those who had come to dedicate their own babies, a woman who had her baby in her hand saw her standing with them without holding a baby in her hand and then gave her own baby to her to carry during the dedication service. She knew that this was the Spirit of God visiting her because they had seen her faith and decided to reward her consistent faith in God for a child. That same year in 2007 she became pregnant after the working of the Spirit of the blessing of the womb and gave birth to *Daniel.* Such acts of faith attract heaven's attention. They are moved by such attitudes of faith, and that is why the Spirit that empowers to become pregnant lighted on her on that day and then succeeded in making barrenness loose its grip on her. Yours is the next release!

**Date:** 24/08/08
**Names:** Mr. & Mrs. I. Babatunde
**Duration:** 4 years of waiting

This couple's testimony attests to the possibility of becoming pregnant with little or no contribution of sperm. Mr. Babatunde shared how they had waited four years to conceive their own baby. One day, he and his wife attended the first service of the night with the King in September 2007 believing that the King has sent for them to meet with them for a change of story. While the service was on and at top gear, **the Bishop started prophesying in the Spirit for a while and then suddenly, the Lord opened the eyes of his wife to see angels of God removing and replacing some things in her tummy and not long, Bishop spoke in English that anyone called barren here tonight shall conceive.** That was it! **"I cannot remember meeting with my wife at all on that day but the scan result showed that she conceived on that same day they returned from the night with the King Service"** he stated. Today, they have given birth to a miracle baby boy named *Copeland, David Oyedepo, Oluwapamileri* (God has made me laugh). Remember, all things are possible if you believe, so begin to focus on the real thing for the formation of your baby in your Womb. Yours is the next testimony!

Date: 27/01/08
Names: Mr. & Mrs. O. Earnest
Duration: Multiple miscarriages ended

The testimony of this couple is really contagious. **According to their testimony, the husband noticed that his wife was suffering miscarriages at every third month of pregnancy. This persisted throughout the year and the husband decided to research the matter because the situation was becoming unbearable for him.** So he told his wife that they needed to ask God what to do to have this plague eradicated, and then they decided to go and see Bishop. Bishop laid hands on her and released the working of the Spirit of the blessing of Sarah upon her, which is the blessing of the womb. **And the Bishop said, "Go and receive your triplets. In case you are afraid, go and take your twins."** Afterwards, she became pregnant and the working of the Spirit of the blessing of the womb ensured that she suffered no more miscarriages. After three months, she went for a scan, and the doctor told her that **the result of the scan revealed that she had just one baby in her womb to which the woman responded, "No way! It has to be two babies in my womb and not one because my Bishop told me to go and take twins in case I'm afraid of having triplet"** The doctor answered that there were actually two but the second one was a fibroid. **Then she answered that it was not a fibroid but a baby, and that she must give birth to her twins notwithstanding what the doctor was seeing.** When it was time for her to deliver she gave birth to twins after the working of the Spirit and today miscarriage, which is the sister of barrenness, has completely loosed its grip on her.

When the working of the Spirit of the blessing of the womb is upon you, you cannot suffer miscarriages. They will not permit it to happen after the order of the working of the Spirit. Therefore, your pregnancy will continue, and you will give birth to your children in the name of Jesus Christ.

Date: 27/04/08
Names: Mr. & Mrs. David O.
Duration: Curse of barrenness dispelled

This couple waited for three years to conceive. There is, however, a remarkable lesson to learn from their testimony. When this couple noticed that children were not forthcoming, the wife opened up to her husband and told him that in her family of origin no women got pregnant. According to her, all her elder sisters who were married before her had not given birth to a baby. **Then the husband answered and said, "You are different, and you will give birth."** The husband told every other person who confirmed what his wife had told him that **his own wife would become pregnant by the working of the Spirit of the blessing of the womb because she was born again and by virtue of marriage to him, she no longer bore the name of her family but instead bore his own name. Thus, he said, whatever curse was working on them would no longer have any effect on his own wife.** They started engaging the light of God's word to fight the curse of barrenness and sow seeds for their unborn children. **They gave names to them and read books on barrenness and the woman kept confessing that she would carry her own children despite whatever curses were prevailing in her family.** Today she is a mother, as she conceived after the order of the working of the Spirit of the blessing of Sarah and gave birth to Jesutofunmi (Jesus is more than enough for me). Did you notice from this couple's testimony that **the man stood his ground rather than fighting his wife or divorcing her to marry another? Men have a lot of role to play in their woman's conception being the authority figure over her life. You have the power to pronounce the blessing of conception on her and possess the authority to invoke the working of the Spirit to bring it to pass.** Remember Genesis 25:21, how Isaac pleaded with the Lord for his wife, Rebekah, and she conceived because the Lord honoured his request? He invoked the working of the blessing of the breast and of the womb on behalf of his wife being the authority over her. I believe embedded in Isaac's plea for Rebecca's conception was for the release of the blessing of conception upon her. It is advised that the man of the house should love to bless his household like David who after blessing the people of Israel would retreat to bless his household (See 2 Samuel 6: 18-20 & 1 Chronicles 16:43). **You are an anointed man; join forces with your wife to make it happen for your family. The words of your children are in your mouth, so begin to speak the blessing until you start talking to them physically.**

Date: 17/08/08
Names: The O. Ajayi's
Duration: 16 years of waiting

Take the example of the Ajayi's, a couple that had being waiting for sixteen (16) years, as a result of their wedding in 1992. Every year, they marked and celebrated their wedding anniversary yet without a child. **Despite this state of childlessness, the** couple continued steadfastly in the service of the Lord in all areas. The lack of a child in their immediate family was not a factor in nurturing the babies of absent parents who were close to them. On a certain day of studying the scriptures, Mr. Ajayi understood the secret of fruitfulness from the gospel according to the book of Luke where God transformed the life of Zechariah, his servant. He realized that the moment he is consistent in his service to the Lord that He shall surprise him the way He surprised Zechariah. The Ajayi's went up to the extent of hosting a home fellowship in their residence, as God revealed the secret of fruitfulness. **They served God consistently and relentlessly believing that someday they would have babies from their own loins.** Then it eventually happened that the wife became pregnant and it was like a dream to them until the doctor confirmed her pregnant. The faithfulness of God, eventually paid-off, the Ajayi's ushered in a twin (boy & girl) on the 8th of August, 2008. This is nothing but the blessing of God and this is an example that God will also remember all your years of waiting and compensate you beyond imagination. You shall be paid-off for those years of waiting for He already called them all blessed who wait for Him (Isaiah 30:18), and He will owe no man. **Be faithful while you are still waiting** for a faithful man shall abound with blessing (Proverb 28:20).

Date: 12/12/08
Name: Mrs. Faith U.
Duration: 14 years of waiting ended

Mrs. Faith had been waiting for her own children for the past fourteen (14) years and had been attending Shiloh. With the encouragement of her pastor, Faith reluctantly attended Shiloh

2007 which is the fourteenth year of her waiting. The servant of God teaching instructed those believing God for the fruit of the womb to write down the names and number of the babies they wish to deliver. Faith stepped forward with the list in belief. In the same month; she noticed a movement in her womb and went for a scan. **After the scan result confirmed she had a tumor with a baby in her womb, the woman chose to believe the words of the blessing that the Bishop had pronounced on her and believed that the power that made her conceive for the first time in fourteen years was capable of sustaining the baby till delivery. That was it!** The state of health of the baby in her hands, when she came up to give her testimony, would show the faithfulness of the promise that only God gives. **The fact that the baby's conception took place outside of the womb, with a tumor resting so close to the baby was not an issue in the development and delivery of her baby.** Who says your powerful baby and fibroid tumors cannot co-exist?

The same power is available waiting for your faith to activate its potential. From this woman's testimony, you will see that the presence of a fibroid tumor in her womb could not hinder the formation of a living being in her womb by the working of the Spirit. **The weed and the wean were allowed to grow together in the same womb to show to us that He cannot be hindered and that He could do it another way, even, in the presence of an enemy towards your childbirth.** Hence, ignore that fibroid because it is not the main issue for your conception to take place. The power of the blessing will render it of none effect to ensure your babies surround your table. You are blessed beyond all curses and fibroid will loose you completely after the working of the Spirit in your womb.

Date: 12/12/08
Name: Mr. Frederick I.
Duration: 11 years of waiting ended

The lack of a child in this family had been persistent for the past eleven (11) years but this did not stop their consistency in attending Shiloh. A doctor's report some years earlier had attributed the infertility in the marriage to a case of low sperm count that the man had been suffering through the years. **The Itula's decided on four children and in faith gave them names as seated around their table, on the instruction from the man of God.** After a short while, his wife conceived, giving birth to a quadruplet in November, 2008. Awesome! **There is just no basis in professional medicine in which a semi-potent man could fertilize his wife of eleven years, with a quadruplet.** The testimony of the Itula's confirms a supernatural working that goes beyond sperm in the fertilization of a baby. The blessing did this for the blessing are upon the head of the just (Proverb 10:6) to undo all that was not so from the beginning.

At the same Shiloh event, I watched live how nothing less than 3,125 children were dedicated to their creator, from mothers who were precisely once tagged barren. They all came out with their babies in their hands and lifted up to heavens in appreciation to the giver of these children. Only God alone could perform all these miracles through the ministry of his son, Dr. David Oyedepo. This is phenomenonal! **All these culminate from the fact that the leader of this ministry takes delight in blessing the people with both the blessing of Abraham and the blessing of Sarah. Do not forget that those who delight in blessing will continually eat of the fruits thereof,** while those who do not will have it far from them (Psalm 109:17). Just like Moses pronounced Naphtali satisfied with favor, and full of the blessing of the Lord (Deuteronomy 33:23), and it was so for him, **so also do the pronouncements of our Spiritual leaders stick to our lives until we become full of the blessing of the Lord.** This ministry and many others who are committed to blessing their sheep and regularly drink the cup of blessing eventually inherit the full blessing of the Lord on earth.

If all these living proof exists in this age and time, then it means God has not changed His style in ensuring that waiting mothers conceive their own children after the workings of the Spirit; therefore, lay hold on the blessings and bother less on your doctor's reports! **Whatever is absent to bring about your conception and delivery is present in His Spirit that works the blessing in you.** Another woman in the same ministry testified **that she conceived even without her two ovaries, which had been surgically removed. Her doctors told her that she would not be able to conceive without ovaries.** The Creator of ovaries, however, who is never short of *spare parts* in His storehouse, chose to display His sovereignty through this woman's situation, and so she became pregnant and the baby developed in her womb and today she is talking to her baby. My eyes almost popped out as I was watching this woman giving her testimony online because she is a *miracle walking on two legs!* Her case so much defied all natural laws regarding pregnancy.

Furthermore, there is also an outstanding testimony on this issue that I came across while watching the messages of Kenneth and Gloria Copeland Ministries online. I have decided to include this testimony because I believe other couples can learn from it and know that age is nothing when it is by the Spirit of life. This couple is one of the KCM partners who attended the Believer's Bible Convention recently and shared their testimony of how barrenness loosed its grip on them. I have documented it below to boost your faith.

Date: 13/03/08
Names: Ruthie & Bob V.
Duration: 14 years of waiting ended

They had been waiting to speak with their children for 14 years without getting a positive result. **According to their testimony, they had attended several meetings and had been prayed for to become pregnant—all to no avail. The wife began to think that they did not need it anymore since they were getting older at 43 years old.** But she began to consider whether she had actually desired to conceive a child in the right way. She realized that her faith was in those prayers and not in God, the Giver of life. Then one day after they moved to Texas, the Holy Spirit showed her Hebrews 11:11, which recounts how Sarah received strength to conceive even in old age. **The woman was prompted to begin to confess that she also received the strength which was the power to conceive even at old age. This became her prayer daily and she believed again that it was possible for her to become pregnant, notwithstanding her age and notwithstanding their doctor's advice to forget about bearing children and go adopt one.** Then, as she continued to confess this scripture, she and her husband attended the Believers Bible Convention in 2007 **and heard Kenneth Copeland teaching that "because God did it for Sarah and for Hannah,** and because He is not a respecter of persons, He would surely do it for you, and so do not doubt it, or even contest it, because you are going to give birth to your own children". Then she realized that this was God confirming the word He gave to her in Hebrews 11:11 through the mouth of Kenneth Copeland. Then she believed that she would bear a child, and today she actually gave birth to her own baby and they are both speaking with their baby now.

This testimony tells us not to give up because of physical depletion arising from ageing or even based on a doctor's diagnosis. This also makes me recall in one of the messages I watched online on the David Oyedepo Ministries website that he mentioned that he had received a letter from a 54-year-old woman who had never had a child saying she had just given birth to her first baby even in her "old age." At her age, many would have given up hope of conceiving, but this woman believed that she was still young enough to conceive and carry a baby in her womb. According to Dr. Oyedepo, this woman would log in and participate in the Shiloh services online and claim for herself all the blessing of the womb released from the mouth of God's prophet, and today she has birthed her own baby at age 54.

Few years ago, I could remember my pastor, Sam Adeyemi, related a story about a couple in Daystar Christian Centre Nigeria who waited over a decade to have children and today have their own baby, their age notwithstanding. By virtue of their relentless attitude of faith they pressed their way out of barrenness. They refused to write themselves off based on their physical circumstances. Do not let anything stop you because your case is not as bad as Sarah. **These can be your own testimony as well if you will stop focusing on your physical deficiencies and focus instead on God's supernatural power. God proved in these women's case that although they were devoid of the necessary biological requirements for conceiving and bringing forth a child, they were not write-offs to Him.** So do not get agitated over that medical report because God knows all about it, and He has not forgotten you but is always right on time.

I read on page 39 in a UK's Sun newspaper dated 16th August, 2008 and written by Emma Morton, a health editor, **how a 70 year old mum gave birth to twins, a boy and a girl in India, even at old age.** This couple have heard two daughters in the past and six grand children **but wanted a male at all cost to inherit their landed properties.** In a bid for a male heir paid for an IVF to give birth to a boy. Having given birth to a boy now, the 77 years old husband exclaimed that he could now die happy and fulfilled. **If at this age, they believed they could still have a son, then your case is not a write off yet. And if this couple did all these just to have a male child to inherit their property after their death, how much more God!** God will do even more within His might and power to see His own heritage come to earth to occupy His place till He comes.

**Dear one, you are too young to retreat–even though you might have waited these many years.** The higher you attain in age while awaiting your children, is a proof that you will have an age long testimony that will tingle the ears of the hearer like that of Sarah's. The blessing of Sarah with Isaac is an age long testimony that stands as a reference point for thousands of years now, and yours is another reference point. So rather than focusing on your flesh and its capacity to conceive, focus on the Spirit that empowers you to become pregnant no matter what fleshly limitations you might have.

**God can suspend the workings of all natural laws in your own case, too,** by releasing the working of the Spirit of the blessing of Sarah on your life, which cannot be thwarted by any mere natural occurrence or medical diagnosis. The working of the Spirit of the blessing of the womb will literally lift you up above all physical obstacles to ensure your conception takes place after the Spirit. **Your conception after the flesh may have been declared impossible but your conception after the Spirit is possible** because it is actually the Spirit who gives life while your flesh is of no profit at all in this matter. Did you see the closing remark of Abraham's biography as accounted in Genesis 24:1? That Abraham died fulfilled because the Lord had blessed him in all things. Is this not the expected kind of fulfillment that He purposes for our end! This is a prototype of the closing remark of your own life as well. You shall have your expected and a fulfilled end by His Sprit working within and walking through life with you in the name of Jesus Christ!

It is finished, said Jesus, and barrenness was not excluded from this statement. Barrenness was finished on the cross years ago, therefore it cannot rule over you for Christ has dealt with it on the cross. Barrenness lost its power over you a long, long time ago. **You will pull through it and have your own seed because it cannot handle a work of the Spirit on your life.** The same way the hardships, decrees, and afflictions of Egypt was not strong enough to withstand the children of Israel from bearing, nothing will stop you either. Whatever curses you may even think is at work will melt before the Spirit of the blessing from the Most High. His blessing will overwhelm and nullify all curses including that of barrenness. **Much more, He would turn the curse into a blessing for you because He loves you so much to sacrifice His son for your freedom.** He has the final say. He could turn and overturn anything to work together for your good. Know that He would prepare a table (of baby Christening) before you, even right in the presence of your enemies. He is not afraid of their tantrums. He would simply make a nonsense of them right before their face and put your dread in them. All that is left for you is to rise up from your cries and worries and walk with your head tall and shoulders high, confident that you are a fruitful being because that is your real status from the very beginning. Therefore, calm down even while you brace up and get ready for the carriage of your children, because you are about to give birth to kings and queens who are the Lord's heritage by the Spirit of the blessing of Sarah working now on your life. **You are the seed of Sarah, and therefore the blessing of Sarah is yours just as the blessing of Abraham is yours.** The breaking news is that the blessing that produced Isaac, Jacob, Joseph, Samuel.. .. John, and Jesus Christ will produce your long awaited babies in your womb.

**You are blessed beyond curses,** and so barrenness in your life is over because the truth of the order of the blessing of the womb has been revealed to you by the help of the Spirit of God. Henceforth, you shall not be named barren anymore because the blessing of Sarah is working on you and in you. You shall die fulfilled like our father Abraham and our mother Sarah because the

Most High will not leave you alone until He has performed this blessing in your life.

*I would recommend that you should purchase the Bible for each of the number of children you anticipate to have and write the names of each of them on it in faith that the owners of these Bibles will come to earth to study and live by it. Remember: acts of faith, pressing into prophetic pronouncements, maintaining right attitudes, seed sowing, positive confessions, personal pronouncement of blessings in prayer, taking care of other people's children and many more acts of service could be means to attract the blessing for conception and a safe delivery.*

# Scriptural Notes

- Genesis 24: 1

- Genesis 25: 21

- Deuteronomy 33: 23

- 2 Samuel 6: 18-20

- 1 Chronicles 16: 43

- Job 14: 7

- Psalm 109: 17

- Proverb 10: 6

- Proverb 28: 20

- Isaiah 30: 18

- Isaiah 54: 1-3

- Habakkuk 2: 3

- Malachi 3: 10

- Ephesians 1: 3

- Hebrews 11: 11

# DIE FULFILLED

Abraham died fulfilled after his wife Sarah receives the blessing for conception. The blessing of Sarah, which is the blessing of the womb, was inevitable for Abraham's fulfillment. Without the blessing of Sarah it was impossible for the joy of Abraham to be full because the blessing of Sarah was the crowning blessing for Abraham and also the fullness of blessings for him since he had everything except an heir. The blessing of Sarah is what made the blessing of Abraham meaningful and the blessing of Sarah is what made Abraham died fulfilled.

Hence his biography shows he was blessed in all things with no exception. The God of our father Abraham saw to it that he and Sarah did not exit the earth childless. He engaged His blessing of the breast and of the womb for Sarah, thus it became impossible for them to die without conception of their own. Similarly, all the couples whose testimonies were shared in this book would inevitably have the same biography as that of Abraham their father, and Sarah their mother because they are already speaking with their children. The common thread in these testimonies is their belief in the Spirit that works out the blessing of the womb in the woman irrespective of their biological knowledge on this matter.

They all at one time or the other received the pronouncement of the blessing of Sarah upon their lives and immediately through faith did settle for its physical manifestation. They did not expect a lesser outcome from what they have discovered about the blessing of the womb. They made sure that barrenness looses them after the God of their father Abraham and mother Sarah aided their flesh to reproduce after its kind.

And mother earth's biography? It cannot be short of dying fulfilled too because she is producing and has not stopped reproducing the entirety of what she was created to conceive till tomorrow. The earth having also experienced a work after the Spirit attained to fulfillment, this should also be your experience Her reproductive cycle is still functional even at old age because she is continually showered with blessing for fruitfulness from heaven. Your biography is taking after these without any iota of doubt. You shall experience the blessing of womb after the working of the Spirit that gives life in you.

He created your womb and every bit of organs responsible for your conception and thus, He alone sees exactly what is required for your baby to be formed in your womb. For this reason, God will bless you with the blessing of Sarah and see through to form your children in your womb despite what is lacking. Your pregnancy shall not be miscarried, you shall give birth to living beings and no child will die in your womb by the Spirit of the God of your mother Sarah. Sarah's body was aged enough to thrust the baby out and her frailty sufficient to make the child die in her womb but her pregnancy and conception was indeed blessed of the Lord.

This is your mother's hall of fame, your own conception and delivery is blessed of the Lord, so no miscarriages for you anymore! And you will not go through the knife to deliver your blessed baby, just as your mother, Sarah did not.

God will strengthen you to pull through and you shall speak with your children on earth. His blood will undertake and avail for you who is facing spiritual battles sustained by ancient altars and covenant. His mercy will speak over judgment in your case, and you shall be redeemed of the Lord, your God. And for everyone striving with fibroid tumors, God will brush through it to form His seeds in your womb. He will cause a clean thing to come out of this unclean thing and you shall conceive notwithstanding. I therefore pronounce you blessed with the blessing of Sarah and yea, blessed indeed to possess a biography of died fulfilled like your father Abraham.

# ACKNOWLEDGEMENT

Firstly, I would like to acknowledge the sources I have been drinking from:

My Spiritual Father and mentor, Pastor Sam Adeyemi, whose encompassing teachings and examples have helped me become an astute believer and a better leader in my journey through life.

My Spiritual Grandfather Bishop David Oyedepo, whose contagious faith and peculiar ministry inspired the writing of this book and has immensely contributed to birthing of many testimonies documented in it through his act of blessing unrepentantly.

Your legend is a blessing to our generation. Thank you sirs!

I am very grateful to my parents; Mr. Joseph and Mrs. Olayinka Owoputi for the patience, love, care, and support shown to me over the years. My siblings are not left out as their constructive criticisms and belief in me have energized and spurred me in life. I love you all.

My many thanks also go to my editing team, Scott Philip Stewart Phd. (USA), Brian Pullinger (UK) and Lanre Briggs (Nigeria) who, inspite of their busy schedules read through this work and made vital inputs. God bless you.

Further, my sincere appreciation goes to some esteemed personalities at the Living Faith World Outreach Ministries Headquarters (HQ) in Nigeria; Pastor Abraham Ojeme, Air Vice Marshal Oluwafemi Ayeni, Daniel Aduloju, and Pastor Taiwo Dixon for their immeasurable support. Thank you!

Many thanks also to all my exceptional friends, within and outside the *Daystar Christian Centre, Lagos,* whose consistent encouragement brought this book to fruition. You are the best!

Ultimately, my special and endless gratitude goes to the Trinity who made it possible for me to undertake this ingenious task. I have enjoyed tremendous grace, love, mercy, and revelation from my King who truly is the source of life.

# About the Author

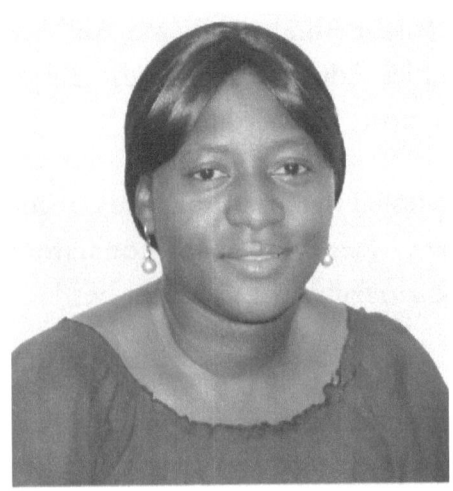

Born in Nigeria, Morolayo is a seasoned Accountant and holds a first degree in Accounting and currently an associate member of the Association of Chartered Certified Accountants (ACCA), United Kingdom, Institute of Chartered Accountant of Nigeria (ACA), and a Certified Risk & Compliance Management Professional (CRCMP), USA. She has had the honour of serving as an auditor in two of Nigeria's most reputable auditing firms; PwC and Deloitte Nigeria, where she brought her accounting skills to bear for almost eight years.

Morolayo is a rare blend of ardour and skill. She also holds a Masters in Economic Governance & Development Management from the University of Birmingham, United Kingdom sponsored by the British High Commission, Department of Foreign & Commonwealth Office in London through the Chevening Scholarship Scheme. She was short-listed based on her fervour for Africa's transformation and her nation's development. She has attended career development trainings in Kenya and Ghana; and also undergone leadership courses at the Lagos Business School (LBS) and the renowned Daystar Leadership Academy (DLA) both based in Lagos, Nigeria.

Morolayo is an astute believer in the fulfilment of womanhood and humanity. She is a lover of God and member of the Daystar Christian Centre, Lagos, Nigeria. Currently, she is garnering more skills for Nation building projects. She resides in Lagos with her family and blessed with a son, Daniel.

# NOTES

- Genesis 17: 16p is Genesis 17: 16 Paraphrased
- KJV: King James Version Reference Bible, copyright ©1994 by The Zondervan Corporation
- NKJV: New King James Version Reference Bible, copyright ©1985 by Thomas Nelson, Inc.

- Dr. David Oyedepo: also being revered as Bishop is the president of Living Faith Ministries, Winners Chapel Worldwide. His mandate is to liberate the world from all oppressions of the devil through the preaching of the Word of Faith.
- Shiloh: is an annual event gathering members of Living Faith Church and believers from all over the world. It has a great spiritual significance and is usually held in December at the Living Faith Ministries Headquarters, Nigeria.
- Testimonies from Faith Tabernacle: were the many testimonies given by members of the Living Faith Church, Worldwide accessed from the ministries' website and used with approval. Available at http://www davidoyedepoministries.org

- KCM: Kenneth Copeland Ministries
- Kenneth Copeland: is the President of Kenneth Copeland Ministries Worldwide. His mandate is to preach the uncompromised Word of God on every available voice and every outreach to meet the needs of people worldwide. The ministries' headquarters is in Texas, United States.
- Believer's Bible Convention: is an event from Kenneth Copeland

Ministries gathering thousands of believers to fully engage them with the Word of Faith and Blessing to change their lives. Testimony shared in this book was from a KCM partner who attended Believer's Bible Convention and accessed from the ministries' website. Available at http://www.kcm.org; 13th March, 2008.

- Sam Adeyemi: is the President of Success Power International and the Senior Pastor of Daystar Christian Centre, Lagos, Nigeria a church with a vision of raising role models. His mandate is to teach scriptural success principles through the media, seminars and publications.
- Watchforce: is the prayer and intercessory unit of the Daystar Church where the Word is enforced to become flesh and work wonders in the lives of many. One of the testimonies shared in this book was an experience of a member of the Watchforce. More information can be accessed at http://www.daystarng.org

- Emma Morton: was the health editor that wrote in the UK's Sun Newspaper, p.39, August 16, 2008 about a 70 year old mum who gave birth to twins in India.

# Let Us Pray

Hannah said, "For this child I prayed, and the Lord has granted me my petition ..." 1Sam 1:27, and so shall the Lord grant your petition for a child as we pray in the name of Jesus Christ;

➤ May the Fertility God lay His hands on you and bless you with the blessing of the breast and of the womb
➤ May He visit you as He visited Sarah, your mother
➤ May He give you the strength to conceive and bringforth
➤ May He impart your humanity with the empowerment for conception, full-time gestation, and safe delivery
➤ May He shower on you His spiritual blessing for fertility from the heavenly places
➤ You shall acquire living beings from the Lord
➤ By His divine fertilizing power, you shall reproduce
➤ May the Lord perform His multiplication agenda to you and fulfill in your life the promise of bearing children
➤ Out of you shall proceed the voice of them that make merry( children)
➤ So far, you have enjoyed addition through marital union, henceforth, you shall enjoy multiplication of humans.
➤ You shall not be put to shame on this matter and the Lord will show you His mercy
➤ May He cause you to conceive in your flesh notwithstanding, and speak with your children after all.
➤ I pray that your baby will not be miscarried nor be thrusted out of its place in the womb
➤ You shall not conceive for sorrow neither shall you bring

forth for trouble

- ➤ May you never experience a painful conception nor sorrowful delivery in the name of Jesus Christ
- ➤ As the Bible records that when the full-time came, Sarah, Elizabeth, and Mary brought forth a son, you, too, shall have a full-time gestation period till you bring forth
- ➤ The Lord, our keeper, will watch over that baby in the dark of the womb, and cause it to take root, bud and blossom till it comes to earth
- ➤ No life shall die in your womb, and may your pregnancy continue
- ➤ He has pronounced your baby blessed, so it shall overcome all forces contending with its arrival to earth
- ➤ May the Lord be your baby's stay in the womb till it emerge a winner against all odds
- ➤ May no power or force be strong enough to bruise the head of your baby in the womb
- ➤ May your womb not be a grave for the life God puts into your womb
- ➤ May He thoroughly prepare and furnish your womb for conception, full-time gestation, and safe delivery
- ➤ May His rivers of living water flush out all obstructions contending with your baby's maturity in the womb
- ➤ May pregnancy not be a disease for you
- ➤ You shall experience the Hebrew women's kind of strength during pregnancy until your delivery.
- ➤ May you experience a trouble free gestation period
- ➤ May you not go through the knife to put your children to bed, rather your children shall descend from your body by His mighty hand

- May His hand turn, and overturn your baby until it maintains the right position in your womb for its safe arrival on earth
- May the fertility God cause all your organs to function properly and work together for your baby's safe delivery
- May your seeds not die in your womb, you shall not have a stillbirth in the name of Jesus Christ
- I pray for you with a confirmed case of fibroid that God's power will turn out a baby from these tumors
- May God raise children to Abraham from these stones
- May He sweep out all the refuge of lies stationed in your womb with His mighty hand
- May His Spirit of burning melt them down for you
- May He prepare a table of baby christening before you in the presence of these enemies called fibroid
- May He cause these tumors to wither away to His own glory.
- Jesus said 'leave the chaff to grow with the wheat' until when the time of separation comes: May He perform this separation for you without the help of man
- May He perform His work, His strange work, and strange act in your case
- May He bring honey out of this rock for you
- May that fibroid turn out a fine boy (girl) for you
- With the help of the Lord, you shall produce a man above all things, and shall acquire a man from the Lord in the name of Jesus Christ.

Welcome to another era of the baby boom!

# Send A Gift

Do you know there is someone out there in your neighborhood, family, office, Church, among friends and loved ones searching for the blessings in this book? Why not reach out today by requesting that a copy of this book in your hand be sent to them as a gift from you.

We can send it on your behalf by simply calling and sending the name(s) and postal address(es) of your recipient(s) with your payment details to +234(0)9020202100 or email morolayo2020@gmail.com

For purchase outside Nigeria, please visit; (www.amazon.com or www.amazon.co.uk, www.authorhouse.co.uk/bookstore) and all other leading bookstore worldwide. Better still, visit the book's website – www.theblessingofsarah.com.

# Also by
# Morolayo Anne Owoputi

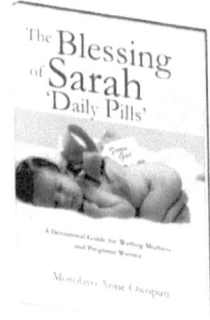

### The Blessing of Sarah 'Daily Pills'

This book is a companion prayer devotional guide to Morolayo Anne Owoputi 'Compelling book' The Blessing of Sarah. It has been designed to help waiting mothers, pregnant women and those with cases of fibroid tumours pray Word-inspired and God-Centred prayers during their devotion. These thirty-one pills if used daily, periodically and overtime, will impact you with power for the impossible and invoke God's blessing on your life for conception, full-time gestation and a safe descending delivery. I see you speaking to your children after all said and done!

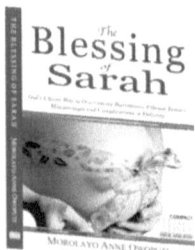

### The Blessing of Sarah Audio Book

The Blessing of Sarah Audio Book comes in a pack of four CDs containing the whole eight chapters of the book. This resource reads the book to you while you are on the move and each of the chapters is arranged in tracks such that you could decide to listen to any chapter of your choice per time. It is a good companion for busy people and for those who wants to keep hearing the Words of Faith until they conceive and birth their babies on earth. You are next in line for a miracle. I see you speaking to your children after all said and done!

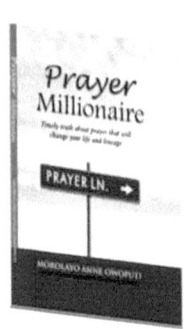

### Prayer Millionaire

This book is fully packed with timely truth on prayer and how you can become a man or woman of prayer effortlessly. It will show you how to cultivate a result-oriented prayer life even in a busy world and how to live a life of abundance in Christ Jesus through revelations and directions flowing out of the fact that you often spend time in His presence. It will definitely fire you up in the belly to pray with focus and surely impact your spirit, soul and body with power to do God's purpose and assignment for your life. Welcome to a new realm with God after reading this book!

*Visit www.theblessingofsarah.com for more information on these books.*